Augmentative and Alternative Communication

HOWARD C. SHANE & MAGGIE SAUER

5341 Industrial Oaks Boulevard
Austin, Texas 78735

The authors wish to thank Harvey Halpern for his continued patience and support during the preparation of this booklet and Sharon Esser for her preparation of the manuscript.

The PRO-ED
studies in
communicative disorders

Series editor
HARVEY HALPERN

Library of Congress Cataloging-in-Publication Data

Shane, Howard C.
  Augmentative and alternative communication.

  (The Pro-Ed studies in communicative disorders)
  Bibliography: p.
  1. Communication devices for the disabled.
2. Speech, Disorders of—Patients—Rehabilitation.
I. Sauer, Maggie. II. Title. III. Series. [DNLM:
1. Communication. 2. Self-Help Devices. 3. Speech
Disorders—rehabilitation. 4. Speech Therapy—methods.
WM 475 S5285a]
RC429.S48   1986   616.85'506   86-16919
ISBN 0-89079-091-4

pro-ed

5341 Industrial Oaks Boulevard
Austin, Texas 78735

10 9 8 7 6 5 4 3 2 1   86 87 88 89 90 91

Contents

Preface

Many individuals experience speech output problems that are so significant that augmented communication methods are required. The purpose of this monograph is to provide a general overview of the field of augmentative and alternative communication. It is an introductory text that includes material on terminology, evaluation, system selection, training methods, and case studies. Additional resources (i.e., augmentative aid descriptions, suggested readings, hardware/software listings) have also been included to provide the reader with information to further complement each of these areas. The content is highly operational and clinically oriented. It emphasizes acquisition, use, and expansion of knowledge in the area of augmentative and alternative communication. While both unaided (e.g., sign language, gestures) and aided (e.g., electronic and nonelectronic aids) communication techniques are included here, emphasis has been placed on the description of aided systems.

Augmentative and Alternative Communication

Terminology

In 1980 the American Speech-Language-Hearing Association published a position statement on augmentative and alternative communication. This paper was designed to provide uniformity with regard to the terminology, standard of service delivery, and personnel training.

A variety of terms have been used to describe communication systems designed for individuals whose speech does not adequately meet communication demands. Terms that have historically been used interchangeably to describe such communication techniques include: nonoral, manual, nonvocal, gestural, nonspeech, nonverbal, alternative, assistive, augmentative, supplementary, aphonic prosthetic, and aided (ASHA, 1980). In each case the terminology describes systems which are designed to supplement a person's existing vocal skills. An augmentative communication system refers to the total functional communication system of an individual and provides a general procedural description which includes both aided and unaided communication.

It is important to distinguish the terms alternative and augmentative when describing communication techniques for the nonspeaking individual. The term *augmentative* denotes techniques which supplement or enhance communication

1

by complementing whatever vocal skills the individual may already possess (Harris & Vanderheiden, 1980b). For some individuals (i.e., severely neurologically impaired), on the other hand, these communication techniques may be viewed as alternatives to speech. The term *alternative* applies when the physical involvement of an individual is so extensive that the production of speech for communication purposes has been ruled out and an alternative communication system is required.

In summary, for the purposes of this text, the term *augmentative communication* will be used as follows: (1) supplementary techniques that enhance communication by complementing whatever vocal skills the individual may possess (Harris-Vanderheiden & Vanderheiden, 1977); (2) any approach designed to support, enhance, or augment the communication of individuals who are not capable of independent verbal communications in all situations (Beukelman, Yorkston, & Dowden, 1985). On the other hand, the term *alternative communication* will be used to describe techniques implemented with individuals when the possibility of communication through speech seems remote and has been ruled out. In other words, in these situations these techniques become an alternative to speech rather than simply complementary.

The importance of making the distinction between augmentative and alternative communication is multifold. For instance, families of persons who are nonspeaking often express concern that a communication aid approach might replace rather than augment speech development or recovery. The term augmentative offers some assurance that the communication goal is to support speech and, in many cases, facilitate its development. The distinction is also important when making clinical decisions with regard to the course of therapy and programming involved in implementing augmentative or alternative methods of communication. Even for the most experienced clinician, however, knowing whether speech will become functional may be difficult at best.

The ASHA position statement suggests that a communication system is comprised of three components: (1) a communication technique; (2) a symbol set or system; and (3) communication/interaction behavior (see Figure 1).

Communication techniques, or the means to transmit concepts or ideas, are divided into two basic categories, unaided and aided. Unaided techniques are those which do not require any physical entity (in addition to one's body) in order to express information. Speech, manual signs or gestures (i.e., sign language, Amerind), and facial communication are all examples of this form of communication transmission. Aided approaches, on the other hand, are those which require some physical medium, object, or device to facilitate the transmission of information. Communication boards, charts, and mechanical/electrical aids are examples of aided communication techniques. Symbol sets or

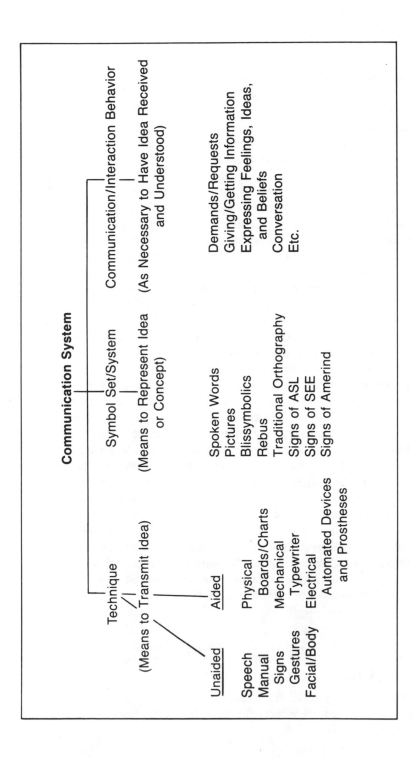

Figure 1. Communication system. From *ASHA* (1980, p. 268).

systems are the means by which ideas or concepts are represented. Spoken words, pictures, Blissymbolics, Rebus, sign language (e.g., American Sign Language, Signing Exact English) are all examples of symbol set/system.

Communication/interaction behavior encompasses some of the more subtle aspects of successful communication transmission. Included are those behaviors deemed necessary to have an idea received and understood. Demanding/ requesting information, giving/getting information, expressing feelings/ideas, and conversational skills (i.e., turn-taking, initiation) are all important in the successful implementation of techniques or systems in a conversational dyad.

Just as the term *augmentative communication* has described a variety of labels, those used to describe the nonspeaking population are equally nonstandardized. Persons who experience severe speech impairments have been labeled nonvocal, nonoral, nonverbal, aphonic, and nonspeaking. Although a severely speech-impaired person can produce some limited speech (and the loss of speech is either permanent or temporary), the residual speech output remains insufficient to meet communication demands. The inability to speak is also independent of hearing impairment (ASHA, 1980). For the purposes of this paper, such an individual will be considered nonspeaking.

Currently, demographic data detailing the size of the nonspeaking population is not well documented, making incidence and prevalence figures speculative. Within the United States there are an estimated 9.9 million persons who have some form of speech impairment (National Institute of Handicapped Research, 1984). Nonspeaking persons were included in these estimates. Within the 9.9 million, 2 million are considered nonspeaking due to a variety of conditions. These estimates were derived from a roll call "guestimate" provided by conference participants. These conditions and their prevalence have been outlined in Table 1. In addition these estimates do not include nonspeaking persons who reside in institutional facilities. For this reason the demographics reported here are felt to be a low estimate of population size. There are over 219,000 mentally retarded persons in residential programs throughout the United States and approximately 119,000 living in state-operated residential facilities. The number of persons who have speech impairments and/or who are nonspeaking within this population has not been clearly delineated.

Characteristics of the Nonspeaking Population

Augmentative and alternative communication approaches are employed with individuals evidencing a variety of conditions. Although the characteristics of each

TABLE 1
Estimated Population of Nonvocal Individuals
in the United States, 1977

Etiology	Prevalence	Nonverbal	Nonvocal
Cerebral Palsy	750,000	10%	20%
CVA Aphasia	1,500,000	50%	50%
ALS	10,000		40%
Multiple Sclerosis	250,000		40%
Parkinson's Disease	4,000,000		10%
Muscular Distrophy	500,000		2%
Laryngectomy	40,000		100%
Deaf	(not included)		
Total, Adults and Children	7,100,000	825,000	1,454,000
Total Children to 16 years (est. × .40)		300,000	581,600

Source: BEH Conference on·Communication Aids for the Nonvocal Severely Physically Handicapped Person, December 7–8, 1976, Alexandria, Virginia.

may differ, they share the feature that speech is neither the most functional nor the primary means of expressive communication. Furthermore, adults as well as children are susceptible to these conditions. Therefore, the age range for which one may expect to find augmentative/alternative forms of communication being used is as diverse as the underlying etiologies.

The following conditions, present at birth, often lead to the prescription of augmentative communication techniques. Congenital abnormalities can be localized or general as well as mild or severe. Prevalence of congenital defects is approximately 3% of live births, but if all abnormalities are included which are discovered the first year of life the rate increases to 6% (Grove, 1976).

Developmental Apraxia

"When certain brain circuits devoted specifically to the programming of articulatory movements are impaired, the resulting articulatory disorder is called apraxia of speech" (Darley, Aronson, & Brown, 1975). Typically individuals who evidence apraxia of speech are unable to accomplish purposeful and volitional motor speech movements, yet may do so in instances of involuntary execution. Some of the characteristics often associated with apraxia of speech include: (1) visible and audible groping as they struggle to produce correct articulatory postures; (2) recognition of errors and effort to correct the error; (3) change in speech rate, stress, and spacing of words in an effort to decrease articulatory errors. Prosody is, therefore, altered as well as articulation (Darley, Aronson, & Brown, 1975).

Each of these characteristics contributes to reduced intelligibility and in some cases leads to the use of augmentative communication techniques. Cohen and Shane (1982) reported that there is a paucity of literature on the use of such techniques with developmental or acquired forms of apraxia of speech. They also suggest a change in the approaches used with this group. Apparently speech-oriented training is being exchanged, at times, for methods utilizing augmentative systems. The authors recommend the application of augmentative procedures when oral speech is not developing, or when response to the treatment is not occurring at a rate which is suitable to prevent the development of frustration or other negative reactions to the communication failure.

Dysarthria

Dysarthria is a collective term used to describe a group of speech disorders resulting from disturbances in muscular control (Darley, Aronson, & Brown, 1975). Because there has been damage to the central or peripheral nervous system, some degree of weakness, slowness, incoordination, or altered muscle tone characterizes the activity of the speech mechanism. This term is also inclusive of coexisting motor disorders of respiration, phonation, articulation, resonance, and prosody.

In children, neurogenic conditions such as cerebral palsy and pseudobulbar palsy give rise to dysarthric speech. Although the degree of impairment may be different in each case, the effect is frequently severe enough to warrant the introduction of an augmentative technique. Intervention strategies often differ for congenital and adventitious forms of dysarthria. The most obvious difference lies in the development of receptive/expressive language competency. For the young child whose receptive and expressive language abilities have not followed the typical developmental process, intervention techniques would, of course, include methods which support normal receptive as well as expressive language development. Cohen and Shane (1982) report that aided systems are most often used to support development of these language skills as well as to augment communication. Harris-Vanderheiden and Vanderheiden (1977) propose additional barriers to communication in the nonverbal severely physically handicapped child aside from those which are obviously related to the physical and motor impairment. These barriers are:

1. Reduced or inconsistent ability to interact with and explore the environment
2. Reduced or inconsistent ability to play/interact with other persons motorically and vocally and to stimulate vocal feedback from caregivers and others
3. Inability to express emotions, needs, thoughts, and to exchange information with others in a consistent, reliable, and effective manner
4. Inability to develop control of "normal" communication mechanisms (oral speech and fine motor mechanisms)

Due to the involuntary motor movement associated with motor disorders such as cerebral palsy, these children are often not recipients of positive environmental stimulation. Situations which are characteristically sources of positive interaction between parent and child may become a source of tension and frustration (Harris-Vanderheiden & Vanderheiden, 1977). Yarrow, Klein, Lomonaco, and Morgan (1975) stated that social stimulation, intensity of expression of positive effect, active kinesthetic stimulation, and variety in the environment are related to cognitive development. The impact of the motor disorder on the child extends beyond that of a mobility and communication problem. Disorders of this nature can lead to cognitive and interactive handicaps which may, in fact, directly inhibit communication development.

Signing and gestural communication systems are often inappropriate strategies for persons who are dysarthric. The restricted fine- and gross-motor movements which often accompany cerebral palsy and other similar conditions make the production of legible signs extremely arduous and nonfunctional for communication purposes. For this reason, aided systems are most often used with persons evidencing dysarthria.

Mental Retardation

Cognitive deficits, particularly the inability to use speech for appropriate interactive exchange, produce conditions in which the implementation of augmentative systems is appropriate. Little information is available regarding the actual number of individuals within this population who use augmentative or alternative means of communication. Cohen and Shane (1980) provide an extensive review of the use of communication systems with the mentally retarded. The studies reported by these authors support the use of both aided and unaided systems to promote successful communication interactions from the mildly to severely retarded person.

The use of augmentative approaches has been reported to facilitate the increase of speech production in severely speech-impaired persons who are retarded. Balick, Spiegel, and Greene (1976), Levett (1969), and Topper (1975) all reported an increase in active communication interaction by their subjects using mime as a communication technique. Silverman (1977) reported an increase in spontaneous communication as well as attempts by subjects to speak when gestures or signing systems were used. Song (1979) taught Blissymbols to severely mentally retarded adolescents. They were able to successfully use the symbols to communicate about items of high preference.

Autism

Autism is manifested at birth or shortly thereafter. Kiernan (1983) provided an overview of the augmentative communication techniques being used with autistic children. He noted that although signing systems were used most often there have been reported cases in which pictographic systems were successfully developed (Carrier, 1976; Light & Remington, 1978). Kiernan concluded that the studies revealed that the use of signs and symbols can mediate more complex language functions by providing a medium for creative and generative language (Kiernan, 1983). A variety of remediation techniques have been used to facilitate language development in the autistic child (Alpert, 1980). It is generally felt that the use of augmentative techniques facilitates general interpersonal communication and speech and can impact noncommunicative behaviors (Cohen & Shane, 1980). Dartnall (1980), Fulwiler and Fouts (1976), Miller and Miller (1973), and Offir (1976) introduced sign language to autistic youngsters as a means of providing them with an expressive communication system. In each case the children were able to use a limited number of signs for functional communication purposes.

Language Disorders

Receptive language deficits can impede normal expressive language development. The inability to encode ideas in conventional syntactic and semantic forms may directly interfere with the normal acquisition and use of speech. Furthermore, deficiencies of this type may interfere with the development of oral speech for functional communication purposes (Ferrier & Shane, 1983). Failure to develop language structures can be attributed to a number of factors which have been mentioned previously, including sensory deficits. Augmentative communication techniques provide a vehicle to support continued language development. The visual and auditory feedback offered through graphic representations and other methods of sensory feedback may permit the user to visually and auditorally organize abstract concepts.

Craniofacial Abnormalities

Severe structural abnormalities can affect the communication process. Congenital structural anomalies (i.e., Apert's syndrome or Treacher Collin's syndrome) vary in the degree of malformation. In some cases, the disfigurement of the facial structures is so extensive that speech becomes highly unintelligible, warranting the introduction of an augmentative communication technique. The communication specialist is cautioned that augmentative techniques can be imposed with this population, but traditional oral speech strategies should not be overlooked.

In contrast to those conditions which are present at birth are those which are acquired or adventitious. The onset of such conditions can be traumatic (e.g., a blow to the head) or progressive, as observed in diseases such as amyotrophic lateral sclerosis or Parkinson's disease. In any case, these individuals are generally linguistically competent or were at one time. The following sections will discuss the application of augmented techniques for once-normal speakers.

Degenerative Neurological Disease

The progressive, degenerative neurological diseases such as amyotrophic lateral sclerosis (ALS), multiple sclerosis, muscular dystrophy, Parkinson's disease, and Huntington's chorea have a special affinity for the speech mechanism. Frequently dysarthria is the speech disorder which results from these conditions and which leads to the need for augmented communication techniques. Aided techniques are more typically used with persons having a motor speech disorder associated with these etiologies. Murphy and Cook (1975) and Sitver and Kraat (1982) describe the use of aided augmentative communication techniques with patients presenting the effects of ALS. Beukelman, Yorkston, and Dowden (1985) report successful use of computer-based scanning systems, manual communication boards, and other alternative writing systems with such conditions.

Cerebral Vascular Accidents

Cerebral vascular accidents often lead to severe motor speech disorders. A variety of methods have been employed in an attempt to optimize communication attempts by these individuals. In some cases speech or prosthodontic treatment have been used to improve intelligibility when there is reason to believe that some function may return to the damaged nervous system (Darley, Aronson, & Brown, 1975). At times, the speech disorder is severe enough to warrant the use of unaided and aided communication techniques. Chen (1971) and Fenn and Rowe (1975) report the use of manual communication systems for dysarthric speakers. Writing and typing have permitted some individuals to augment communication attempts but are often insufficient due to the physical limitations which are present, thereby reducing speed and legibility. Communication boards have been designed for use with linguistically intact persons. Beukelman and Yorkston (1977) describe a communication technique designed to maximize communicative effectiveness by combining verbal communication with a spelling system (letter cueing) on an alphabet-number board. Other attempts to augment communication with aided techniques have been reported by Buzolich (1981); Beukelman and Yorkston (1982); and Beukelman, Yorkston, and Dowden (1985).

Aphasia

Aphasia is a condition which frequently results from cerebral vascular accidents. When there is an "impairment in the cerebral hemisphere that has as its primary function the processing of the language code, the resulting language disorder is aphasia. Aphasia is a multimodality reduction in capacity to interpret and formulate meaningful linguistic elements. It is manifested in difficulties in listening, reading, speaking, and writing" (Darley, Aronson, & Brown, 1975, p. 5). Aphasic individuals differ from individuals afflicted with a congenital disability because their need for augmentative or alternative means of communication may change after the initial posttrauma period. In these cases communication treatment may include augmentative/alternative techniques which are temporary or perhaps permanent in nature. Furthermore, since the aphasic person's linguistic competency may evolve over time, communication needs also change. Little research has been done with regard to the application of augmentative communication techniques with aphasic patients (Cohen & Shane, 1982). Response to augmentative communication techniques is unclear. Beukelman and Yorkston (1982) and Beukelman, Yorkston, and Dowden (1985) discuss the successful implementation of aided systems with aphasic clients. Other studies by Estabrooks and Walsh (1985) found that aphasics' communication did not improve. This suggests that aphasia is a pervasive language disorder. Those studies reported by Beukelman and Yorkston (1982) and Beukelman, Yorkston, and Dowden (1985) provide a more optimistic outlook. Communication books, gestures, and automated communication devices were among those techniques used to augment communication attempts.

Head Injury

Head injuries sustained from external sources such as automobile accidents, gunshot wounds, or blows to the head often lead to a motor speech disorder.

Residual communication skills may vary from anarthria to mild speech or linguistic impairment. Similarly little has been reported on the use of augmentative communication techniques with the head-injured population. Microcomputer-based systems (Beukelman, Yorkston, & Dowden, 1985) as well as simple non-electronic communication boards (DeRuyter & David, 1982) are among the aided systems reportedly used.

Anatomical Anomalies

Conditions resulting in the surgical removal of part or all of the anatomical structures (e.g., glossectomy, laryngectomy) necessary for speech production provide situations in which an augmented technique may be used. Glossectomy or the removal of part or all of the tongue may, in some cases, make speech an impossibility. Similarly, surgical excision of the larynx and associated anatomical structures necessitates the implementation of artificial laryngees, esophageal speech, or other aided and unaided techniques.

Hospitalized patients in intensive care units (ICU) are among the individuals who present with conditions which do not permit the successful transmission of communication. Tracheostomies are often performed on ICU patients to provide respiratory assistance. Other mechanical methods of medical treatment also interfere with the successful production of speech, thereby suggesting the feasibility of an augmented technique.

Overview of Communication Techniques and Systems Access

The decision on how to best facilitate communication in handicapped persons is heavily dependent upon their physical abilities. In order to construct messages using graphics or orthographic symbols, a method of selection must be designed which permits the individual to indicate selections as quickly and easily as possible. There are three basic methods of indication. These include scanning, encoding, and direct selection.

Scanning is defined as "any technique (or aid) in which the selections are offered to the user by a person or display, and where the user selects the characters by responding to the person or display. Depending upon the aid, the user may respond by simply signaling when he sees the correct choice presented, or by actively directing an indicator (e.g., light or arrow) toward the desired choice" (Vanderheiden & Harris-Vanderheiden, 1976, p. 21).

Examples of scanning techniques include the use of a communication board while a second person points to each symbol, word, or letter until the desired character is pointed to, or use of a single switch that directly signals an aid when the desired character is reached by a marker on the display. There are six basic types of scanning motions which one may select in order to provide the most effective means of indication. They are linear, stepped, row/column, directed, latched, and predictive scanning:

1. *Linear scanning.* When a marker or indicator sequentially moves from the top left-hand corner of a display to the bottom right-hand corner. One button/switch activation will cause the moving indicator to stop and a second will cause it to start over. Because the linear scanning techniques can be extremely slow, alternative scanning techniques were developed in order to decrease the time required to select target message components.

2. *Stepped scanning motion.* When the indicator or marker proceeds successively from one target to the next. Each activation of the button/switch causes the indicator to move to the next target.

3. *Row/column scanning motion.* The indicator or marker will display each row in succession. When the button/switch is activated, the indicator will scan across the row one frame at a time until the anticipated column is reached. The next switch activation will cause the indicator to stop at the chosen frame. Another button/switch activation causes the scanning operation to start again.

4. *Directed scanning motion.* A control device such as a joystick can be used to move the indicator up, down, left, right, or diagonally. A button/switch activation will fix or stop the display at its current position.

5. *Latched scanning motion.* In the stepped scanning mode, a button or switch can be depressed which will cause the indicator to scan automatically. When the switch is released, the scan motion is terminated.

6. *Predictive scanning motion.* A technique commonly used in computer-aided scanning. Selections are made from the letters of the alphabet as the indicator or marker moves through the display. When a selection is made, the aid tries to "predict" which character will be selected next. The characters which have a high predictive value to be selected are then presented. If the intended selection is not contained within the characters presented, the original scanning sequence is resumed. Although this technique is limited to scanning arrays with alphabetic displays, it can increase the rate of selection significantly, thereby increasing communication rate.

Scanning techniques can be particularly powerful because they can be implemented with severely physically handicapped individuals. These techniques require only that an individual have a voluntary movement which can signal a communication partner or communication device that a selection has been made. The means by which a device can be signalled is through a single switch activation. The switch that implements this function is controlled by the individual's movement and can be selected from a variety of switches to take best advantage of the movement or response (see Appendix E). Persons who have low cognitive abilities can operate and use these techniques with relative ease.

The greatest disadvantage of scanning methods is the time required to construct and transmit messages. The user as well as the communication partner must wait as the indicator moves through the display each time a selection is made.

Encoding is a technique designed to increase rate of message selection. Encoding is defined as follows: "The desired choice is indicated by a pattern or code of input signals, where the pattern or code must be memorized or referred to on a chart. When an aid is used, any number of switches may be used. The code may involve activating the switch, sequentially or simultaneously" (Vanderheiden & Harris-Vanderheiden, 1976, p. 22).

One example of an encoding system would be a color-coded eye gaze system. The user indicates that his selection is contained within a particular cluster of pictures located on an eye gaze chart, through eye gaze. The target symbol within the cluster is then selected in the same manner just described, by selecting the corresponding color of the target symbol from an array of colors. Morse code or some other code can be used in conjunction with a single switch. The coded items can then be decoded and displayed on a television monitor or reproduced on a typed display.

Encoding techniques can decrease the time needed for message construction because they can increase the speed with which selections can be made. These techniques require higher cognitive abilities, however, than scanning or direct selection. In addition, displays used with traditional scanning techniques often become limiting due to the number of characters which can be provided on the display. Encoding permits the user to retrieve vocabulary from more than one display, thereby increasing vocabulary availability. For example, a display may contain only numerals. However, numeric codes can be developed which correspond to vocabulary contained on a separate listing. In this way, a relatively large vocabulary can be used and increased simply by selecting numeric codes from a numeric scanning display.

Direct selection is the easiest and fastest of all selection techniques. It is "any technique (or aid) in which the desired choice is directly indicated by the user. In direct selection aids there is a key or sensor for each possible choice or vocabulary element" (Vanderheiden & Harris-Vanderheiden, 1976, p. 26).

Pointing to letters or symbols on a communication board is an example of the direct selection technique. This method of selection is not only common to manual communication boards but many of the automated communication aids as well. It provides a straightforward means of indicating those components used to construct messages for communication. The visual cues provided by the display are particularly helpful for persons presenting low cognitive ability. For the physically able, direct selection is the quickest, most efficient means of indication.

There are a considerable number of commercially available communication systems designed to meet a variety of needs. The naive consumer may at first be overwhelmed by the number of systems available and find it difficult to come to any conclusions with regard to system capabilities, function, and the differences between each. Nearly all systems possess three basic components which allow the consumer to begin to classify them. Beukelman, Yorkston, and Dowden (1985) identify them as system control, process, and output.

System control refers to the display and interface. The display is what the user observes when operating the system. Panels containing letters, numbers, lights, symbol systems, and combinations thereof are all displays. Displays can include the keyboard on a typewriter or a panel divided into target areas containing infrared light detectors. Characters included on the display range from symbol representations to traditional orthographic representations.

Determination of how to best interface an aid is based upon the individual's physical abilities. Severely physically involved individuals may use a scanning system whereby a single switch is the interface used to make selections from a display. Direct selection interfaces are an option for the less physically impaired.

The function performed by the system is known as the *system process.* There are three types of processes typically seen in commercially available communication systems. The first are those systems which do not store or decode information but simply transmit it. An example of such a system is a conventional typewriter. Use of the keys corresponding to a letter of the alphabet results in printing of that letter only. Retrieval of coded information is the second process. This coded information may be letters, words, or phrases and is retrieved by activating a code. As Beukelman, Yorkston, and Dowden (1985) note, some devices can be purchased with vocabulary which has been preprogrammed by the manufacturer, considered here fixed vocabulary. Other aids can be programmed by the user as their needs and environment dictate. The third process is the preparation, storage, and retrieval of information by selecting a single "routine." Messages prepared in advance may significantly increase the rate of communication interaction.

The third major component of a communication system is the *output*. Visual output and auditory output systems are the most common types of output in communication aids. Printers, typewriters, and television screens are all examples of visual output. Devices in which the display is spoken via a speech synthesizer or human voice (e.g., digitized speech, tape recorder) are examples of auditory output.

Communication Techniques

It is apparent that communication can be augmented by many techniques. The complexity of these techniques ranges from nonautomated systems that do not require the use of a physical aid (e.g., sign language, Amerind) to fully automated microcomputer systems that can provide an individual with a means to independently communicate and accomplish writing tasks. Automated or nonautomated communication systems can be classified according to their function:

1. Unaided communication systems
2. Nonelectronic communication aids
3. Electronic communication aids (dedicated or multipurpose)
4. Microcomputer systems using dedicated communication software

The third and fourth categories are descriptions of "dedicated" communication aids and software. In other words, the operational function of these aids is to provide a means of expressive communication. A dedicated aid uses synthesized speech or text as the vehicle for communication but does not possess other functions which enable the individual to complete educational or vocational writing tasks, control the environment, or use the phone. They do, however, produce messages which can be constructed to suit the user's needs, stored for future use, or used for immediate communication. The VOIS 130, 135, and 140 produced by Phonic Ear are all examples of dedicated communication devices (see Appendix F for more detailed information).

Unaided Communication Systems

Unaided systems of communication are techniques which do not require any external communication aid. Examples of unaided systems are American Sign Language, signing Exact English, and Amerind. Signing and gestural systems provide a method of communication for a broad range of disabled persons but typically those having a span of intellectual abilities, autism, hearing impairment, and mild physical impairment. Factors which should be considered before assigning the task of learning one of the aforementioned communication techniques might include: (1) sufficient fine-motor skills that will support the production of visibly intelligible signs or gestures, and (2) sufficient environmental support for parents, spouses, and peers to be able to interpret and use the signs or gestures. These systems tend to be exclusive because of the knowledge required by all interactants to use and interpret this communication medium. As such, the number of people who interact with the user may be restricted.

Aided Communication Systems

Nonautomated communication aids have no electronic parts. Typically these aids are constructed using photographs, picture symbol systems (i.e., Picsyms, Bliss, Rebus, or Mayer-Johnson picture line drawings), the alphabet orthographic representations consisting of words and phrases, or combinations thereof. Nonautomated or nonelectronic communication aids are a versatile form of communication. Because of the ease of construction, parents, teachers, and spouses can conceivably design and construct nonautomated devices. The actual vocabulary content for the aid should suit the nonspeaking person's individual needs. This is extremely important as it provides all communication interactants, readers and nonreaders alike, with an interpretable form of communication. Nonspeaking persons with reading skills may use a board containing words and phrases similar to the one in Figure 2. On the other hand, someone who does not have the ability to read may possibly use a system like the one in Figure 3, which contains picture symbols. Generally, nonautomated systems can provide a direct and effective method of communication for the mildly physically handicapped person as well as the mild to severely mentally retarded.

While nonautomated systems can provide a means of communication for a variety of nonspeaking persons, they may not solve all the person's communication needs. Most often direct selection is a very difficult, if not impossible, task for the severely physically disabled. Use of a nonautomated system can be accomplished if a second person acts as a "scanner" moving through the display naming each character. This is, of course, an ineffective means of communicating because of the time it requires to complete a message and the concentration required by all interactants during the exchange. During such an interaction, the communication partner assumes responsibility for the flow and interpretation of the exchange by carefully recording each message element as it is selected. In addition, the area required to record additional vocabulary items increases commensurate with expanding vocabularies. Without a more efficient means of organizing and storing vocabulary, the size of a nonelectronic com-

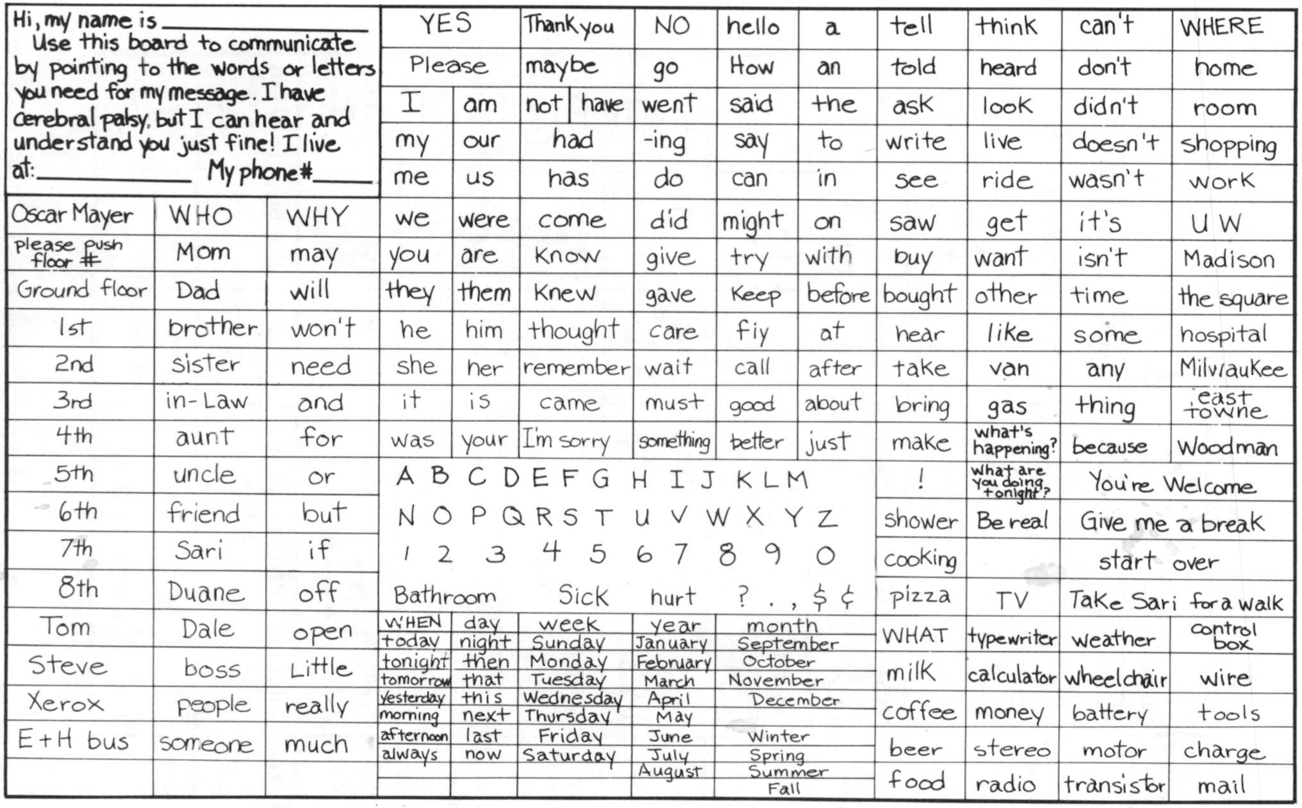

Figure 2. Alphabetic communication aid.

Instruction block (top left):

Hi, my name is _____
Use this board to communicate by pointing to the words or letters you need for my message. I have cerebral palsy, but I can hear and understand you just fine! I live at: _____ My phone# _____

Left directory / WHO / WHY columns:

	WHO	WHY
Oscar Mayer	Mom	may
Please push floor#	Dad	will
Ground floor	brother	won't
1st	sister	need
2nd	in-Law	and
3rd	aunt	for
4th	uncle	or
5th	friend	but
6th	Sari	if
7th	Duane	off
8th	Dale	open
Tom	boss	Little
Steve	people	really
Xerox	someone	much
E+H bus		

Main word grid:

YES	Thank you	NO	hello	a	tell	think	can't	WHERE
Please	maybe	go	How	an	told	heard	don't	home
I / am	not / have	went	said	the	ask	look	didn't	room
my / our	had	-ing	say	to	write	live	doesn't	shopping
me / us	has	do	can	in	see	ride	wasn't	work
we / were	come	did	might	on	saw	get	it's	U W
you / are	Know	give	try	with	buy	want	isn't	Madison
they / them	Knew	gave	keep	before	bought	other	time	the square
he / him	thought	care	fiy	at	hear	like	some	hospital
she / her	remember	wait	call	after	take	van	any	Milwaukee
it / is	came	must	good	about	bring	gas	thing	east towne
was / your	I'm sorry	something	better	just	make	what's happening?	because	Woodman

---

Letters:

A B C D E F G H I J K L M
N O P Q R S T U V W X Y Z

Numbers:

1 2 3 4 5 6 7 8 9 0

Punctuation / symbols: ? . , $ ¢

Phrases / objects (lower grid):

You're Welcome · Give me a break · Be real · start over · Take Sari for a walk · what are you doing tonight? · ! · shower · cooking · pizza · TV · Bathroom · Sick · hurt

tell	think	can't	WHERE
WHAT	typewriter	weather	control box
milk	calculator	wheelchair	wire
coffee	money	battery	tools
beer	stereo	motor	charge
food	radio	transistor	mail

Time:

WHEN	day	week	year	month
today	night	Sunday	January	September
tonight	then	Monday	February	October
tomorrow	that	Tuesday	March	November
yesterday	this	Wednesday	April	December
morning	next	Thursday	May	
afternoon	last	Friday	June	
always	now	Saturday	July	
			August	

Seasons: Winter · Spring · Summer · Fall

me /my /11+	you	we	are, is, am	fix	hold me	put away
Pam / Karin	Mom	woman	be	forgot	hope	read
Judy / Red	Dad	man	believe	get	itches	see
Bob	boyfriend	baby	brush	give	like	sew
Sheila Ann	friends	boy	change clothes	go, walk	love	sit
Dennis Aide	doctor / dr	girl	close	gossip	lying	sleep
foster parents	lawyer	O.T.	come	got	married	stop
him / her	social worker	P.T.	drink	hate	need	suppose
police	relative	Speech therapist	eat	have	open	take
people	wife	husband	fall	help	pick up	talk/tell say/said
nobody	bitch	Hans Kasten 555-2083	divorce	cry	hide	kiss

Figure 3. Nonalphabetic communication aid.

tear off	want	who	afraid	funny	new	bossy
think	tease	what	awful	good	nice	fun/enjoy
thought	ask	when what time	bad	happy	old	sense of humor
touch	cope, can	why	care	hard	sad	Irish green inside
trimmed	do	where	crazy	hurt	same	cold
watch	feel	How	damn	jealous	sick	hot/warm
wash	find	know	depressed	left out	slow	bored
wait	chip in	adjust	different	mad	stupid	beautiful
wish	memory remember	moving	easy	mean	tall, big	too babyish
work	borrow	can't not /don't	fair	moody	upset	shocked
introduce	break in	try	free	neat	wierd	worried

Figure 3. Continued.

munication aid can be voluminous. Electronic devices were developed to meet these needs by providing "programmable storage areas" to store vocabulary, which can then be saved for future use. Furthermore, certain electronic aids were designed to meet not only communication needs but to assist the physically handicapped in becoming more educationally and vocationally independent. Text production and editing and environmental control functions are only a few of the features available in some of the automated systems of today.

Electronic communication aids vary in their function and complexity. It is most helpful to classify electronic communication aids as dedicated or multipurpose and portable or nonportable.

Dedicated communication devices are those systems which are exclusively designed to furnish an augmentative alternative means of communication through spoken or written output. Characteristically, spoken output is produced in the form of synthesized speech, and written output is produced on small displays or printers located internally or externally to the system. Dedicated aids can also be classified as portable or nonportable. Portable aids are systems which can move from place to place with the user. It is not restricted to one environment due to power system needs or size. Rather, they can operate in various settings because they are not dependent on external power sources for operation (Vanderheiden & Harris-Vanderheiden, 1976). Examples of dedicated communication devices are the VOIS 130, 135, 140 from Phonic Ear, the Epson Speech Pak, and Vocaid from Texas Instruments, to name a few (see Appendix F).

Multipurpose communication devices are designed to meet the communication needs served by dedicated systems but also to perform additional operations such as environmental control (e.g., turning lights and household appliances on and off). They can be interfaced to a microcomputer system for standard computer operation. Similarly, multipurpose devices can be classified as portable or nonportable depending on whether or not they are independent of external power sources. Examples of multipurpose portable systems are the Express III, Light Talker, Touch Talker, and Minspeak from Prentke Romich Company as well as the Trine System developed by the Trace Center of Madison, Wisconsin. The Words+ Living Center, produced by Words+ in Sunnyvale, California, is an example of a nonportable multipurpose system (see Appendix F).

Microcomputer systems using dedicated communication software developed with the advent of smaller, more portable general-purpose microcomputer systems and the use of software written and developed exclusively for the nonspeaking population. Once again, the term *dedicated* in this case denotes software used with a microcomputer system to supplement communication through spoken output. Spoken output is accomplished through synthetic speech produced by a speech synthesizer. These software programs allow the user to select messages for communication by selecting keys on the computer keyboard or activating a single switch. Much like their dedicated communication aid counterparts, dedicated software programs permit the user to select messages from preprogrammed vocabulary menus or programs and store their own vocabulary contents for future retrieval. Additionally, software programs are often available with a number of different options to accommodate the abilities of the user. For instance, if the user is unable to use a program which requires direct selection from the keyboard, scanning options may be available which have single switch modifications. Hard-copy text production is another feature often included in these software packages. In other words, should the user choose to print a message in hard-copy form via an external printer rather than spoken output, he or she can select to do so. A standard microcomputer system can be modified for dedicated communication software by simply interfacing the system with a speech synthesizer.

Using dedicated communication software with a general-purpose microcomputer system presents a number of advantages. First of all, software programs can be developed which can accommodate the needs of a wide range of individuals with varying cognitive and physical abilities. In many cases the non-speaking population has needs in their environment which require the use of microcomputer systems—needs which are not served by other communication devices. Adaptive software permits the handicapped person to communicate on and perform other vocational and education tasks using one system. Thus the microcomputer can assume a role in communication in addition to other roles it standardly serves. (See Appendix G for dedicated communication software listings.)

Standard computer access is another important communication technique. Utilizing the computer as a work and communication tool often requires modifications to allow the physically handicapped person to access or control the computer. These modifications, which can be made directly to the keyboard or the actual computer hardware, allow disabled persons to manipulate computer functions.

The most common example of keyboard modification is a keyguard placed over the keyboard. Keyguards are shields with holes over each key which permit the user to select one key at a time without unintentionally depressing other undesired keys. Commonly used computer commands requiring the simultaneous activation of two keys can also be executed with the aid of a keyguard because of the built-in latching mechanism. The keyguard is particularly useful

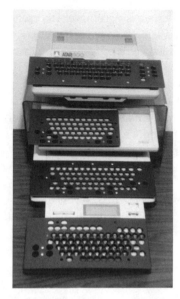

Figure 4.   Keyguards. Courtesy of Prentke Romich Co.

with individuals presenting spastic or athetoid cerebral palsy. Figure 4 contains an example of a keyguard.

Keyboard emulators are another alternative to standard keyboard access. Emulators offer alternative input modes for entering information into and controlling the computer. This term simply means that the emulating device makes the computer "think" that its own keyboard is being used to enter information or control its operations. In effect, alternative external devices can then be connected to the computer which will then act in place of the keyboard to control standard computer operation. The emulator itself is a small circuit card which is placed in the computer with little modification. The Express III, Touch Talker, Light Talker, Minspeak, and Trine System all previously described can be interfaced with a microcomputer system as alternate keyboards with a keyboard emulator.

In some instances, the implementation of an emulator is unnecessary. Expanded keyboards are another viable alternative. Expanded keyboards are constructed in a variety of designs which more suitably accommodate the needs of a particular individual, such as increased key size, key placement, and user-adjustable key response time.

Still another method of computer control is the single switch. It can be interfaced with the computer through simple adaptations to a joystick to permit a single-switch user to play computer games or make choices from a scanning array.

An Overview of Evaluation and Training

The Importance of Communication

Because communication occurs so naturally and spontaneously most people give little thought to its importance in their daily lives. McDonald (1980) describes communication as a unifying function that takes place among persons who group themselves together to form a community. The communication deficits of the nonspeaking can potentially interfere with community involvement and interaction. It is nearly impossible to estimate the influence of the community in our lives. Beyond the opportunities it provides for communication, it is a vehicle for social interaction and personal development. With a simple request or statement it is possible to alter our environment (e.g., requesting an object, asking a question, expression of emotion). Nonspeaking persons, unfortunately, often appear to be very passive and unmotivated in their interaction with others. It should not be forgotten, however, that physically disabled individuals do not have the same opportunity to interact with the community as physically able persons do. Thus they continue to be viewed as persons who have come to be and are content in being dependent on the community. Perhaps this is because they are not, and don't know what it means to be, a member of their community (McDonald, 1976).

Language Acquisition

Maturation of expressive and receptive language skills is dependent on the ability to organize and act upon one's environment. In other words, individuals must possess the physiological resources which allow them to extract/process information from their surroundings. For the severely physically handicapped person "normal" receptive language development can be attained in a supportive atmosphere through alternative methods of language stimulation. The beginnings of language development can be traced back to the mother/child interaction. As previously noted (McDonald, 1976), the normal communication exchange between a mother and child is strengthened by the positive product of such an exchange: the coos, smiles, and laughter. Since this exchange is not easily produced with the physically impaired infant, it is reasonable to assume that the interaction may not be positively reinforcing for the parent. The result is less interaction and language experience for the child.

McDonald (1976) states that early experiences provide the foundation for later development:

> The interactions which take place during the time of maturation and learning give rise to experiences, the first of which are very simple. The child merely senses that something is occurring. It may be that he hears something or doesn't hear anything. He feels something, he doesn't feel anything. A little later he begins to notice that there are differences in these sensations and at that point he is discriminating between stimuli. He later begins to develop perception by adding to these discriminative sensations some interpretation: mother's voice, father's voice, the dog barking. A little later he will generalize his perceptions into concepts—the building block of language. (p. 7)

Benefits of Augmentative/Alternative Communication

Augmented techniques can enhance cognitive/linguistic development by facilitating cognitive representational skills (Musselwhite & St. Louis, 1982). This notion agrees with current thought on the development of oral language production to augment communication (Vanderheiden & Harris-Vanderheiden, 1976) to enhance oral intelligibility (Beukelman & Yorkston, 1977). Silverman (1980) concluded that "...intervention with nonspeech communication modes can be rationalized for the purpose of speech facilitation as well as improving message transmission" (p. 4). He also concludes that these modes can increase attention skills as a result of two simultaneous sensory inputs: auditory and visual stimuli. Furthermore, the auditory and visual combination provides a more concrete means of representing and organizing language. For the oral but sometimes unintelligible speaker it affords a means of clarifying unintelligible speech. For the nonspeaking individual, active participation in the community and society requires that they continue to communicate with peers, teachers, employers, children, and spouses. Using an augmentative system increases the probability that these opportunities will continue to be possible.

Musselwhite and St. Louis (1982) provide a list of advantages and disadvantages of nonvocal output modes compared to vocal output modes in Table 2. The table also presents a number of disadvantages inherent in the use of augmentative or alternative forms of communication. Most often the disadvantage is found in the expense of these systems or the acceptance of these systems in work, home, or school environments. These issues will be addressed in more detail later.

TABLE 2
Advantages and Disadvantages of Nonvocal Systems
(as Compared to Vocal Systems)

Advantages	Disadvantages
1. Nonvocal systems provide two simultaneous inputs (e.g., auditory and visual).*	1. Nonvocal systems are not typical systems of communication and may not be as readily reinforced by vocal language users.
2. Nonvocal systems have not been found to inhibit development of vocal language; in fact, a number of studies suggest that nonvocal systems may enhance speech and/or language development (see Silverman, 1980).	2. Persons in the environment may be hesitant to accept use of a nonvocal system, as they may feel it represents giving up on vocal language.
3. Nonvocal systems may serve various purposes relative to vocal language: a. Interim communication system (thus may reduce frustration level); b. Speech and/or language facilitation; c. Supplement to vocal language; d. Ultimate communication system.	3. Persons in the environment may be unable to receive the message (e.g., may not know sign or Blissymbols).
4. Nonvocal systems are typically more static, which should help in learning (that is, each entry is available longer).	4. Persons in the environment may not be willing to take the time necessary to receive messages.
5. Nonvocal systems are often more amenable to physical prompting (e.g., the client can be taken through a sign or the gesture of pointing to a symbol).	5. Nonvocal systems may be more expensive due to the need to buy equipment and/or to train persons to teach and receive the message.
6. Nonvocal systems may be slowed down more than vocal language, with less distortion.	

* Although there is some visual input in vocal language, it is not as intense or lasting as in nonvocal language.

Source: Musselwhite and St. Louis (1982, p. 28).

Considerations for the Evaluation of Nonspeaking Persons

The decision to recommend augmentative communication systems has widespread effects for the system user as well as all other communication interactants. For this reason careful consideration must be given to the decision process leading to election of an augmentative form of communication. Several authors (Chapman & Miller, 1980; Harris & Vanderheiden, 1980; Harris-Vanderheiden & Vanderheiden, 1977; Shane & Bashir, 1980) have suggested a number of factors relevant to the decision process. Shane and Bashir (1980) have formalized this process by creating a branching decision matrix, which is presented in Figure 5.

Although the election decision matrix can serve as a clinical aid, the decision process continues to require clinical art as well as a clinical science base (Cohen & Shane, 1982). This prescribed system of evaluation provides documentation of the process and lends support to an "intuitive clinical decision" by systematically outlining a process for parents, teachers, and clients. Moreover, it does not require an individual to move through each of the 10 categories of assessment. Rather, parts of the matrix become inappropriate for certain clients because of the etiologies they present. The decision to immediately implement an augmentative communication system with the occurrence of persistent oral reflexes (movement from Level II to Level X) is exemplary of this.

The decisions generated from the matrix are specified as to whether the final decision is to elect, delay, or reject an augmentative communication system. A decision to elect indicates that the system will be used to facilitate oral language production, augment communication, enhance oral speech intelligibility, or some combination of the above (Shane & Bashir, 1980). A decision to delay indicates that an augmentative communication system is inappropriate at the time, possibly because of lack of cognitive readiness or the need to study the effects of a different form of therapy. A decision to reject indicates that expression via speech rather than through an augmented technique system is considered more appropriate.

The decisions generated from the matrix are specified as to whether the final decision is to elect, delay, or reject an augmentative communication system. A decision to elect designates that such a system be used to facilitate oral language production (Skelly, Donaldson, & Fust, 1973), to augment communication (Vanderheiden & Harris-Vanderheiden, 1976), to enhance oral speech intelligibility (Beukelman & Yorkston, 1977), or some combination of the above. A decision to delay indicates that an augmentative communication system is inappropriate at the time, possibly because of lack of cognitive readiness or the need to study the effects of a different form of therapy. A decision to reject indicates that expression through speech rather than through a nonspeech system is considered more appropriate.

The decision matrix consists of the 10 categories (Levels I–X), the specific components of each category, and the branching alternatives (see Figure 6).

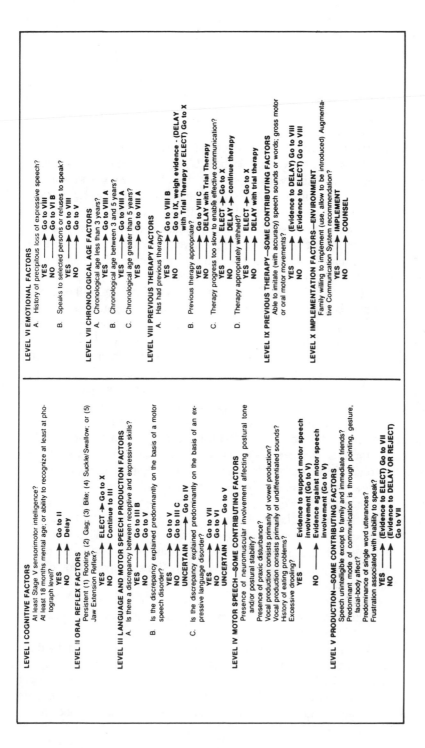

Figure 5. The decision matrix. From Shane and Bashir (1980, p. 409).

Level I Cognitive Factors. At the first level, cognitive factors are investigated. The three specific interrelated factors deal with sensorimotor intelligency (Chapman & Miller, 1980), mental age, and the ability to represent through pictures (Shane, 1980). Noncompliance with any of these factors leads to a decision to delay. Such a decision reflects the lack of cognitive prerequisites necessary for intentional communication (Chapman & Miller, 1980; Reichle & Yoder, 1979) or the ability to represent the object world through two-dimensional pictorial information. In this case, attention to facilitating cognitive growth, such as that advocated by Kahn (1978), is recommended. Moreover, teaching specific prerequisite abilities for augmentative communication system use might be suggested — that is, attending behavior, scanning, direct selection, and/or visual discrimination. Compliance with one or more of the cognitive factors leads to Level II, a focus on oral reflex factors.

Level II Oral Reflex Factors. A significant aspect of the oral reflex level of the decision matrix is that, of all the factors investigated, obligatory persistence of oral reflexes can, in isolation, lead to a decision to elect an augmentative communication system. No other factor in isolation has such a solitary influence on election. Our observation and that of others experienced in prespeech intervention and speech therapy for the cerbral palsied (Mysak, 1963) is that persistent pathological oral reflexes suggest an extremely poor prognosis for oral speech development. We view these factors as an early predictor of failure to develop speech and as one which leads to election of an augmentative communication system. Thus, if these factors are present, a move to Level X Implement Factors — Environment is recommended. In addition, the recommendation to try to inhibit the obligatory reflex patterns might be appropriate. The nonexistence of abnormal oral reflexes leads to Level III.

Level III Language and Motor Speech Production Factors. This level is used to establish whether motor (Level III B) or language (Level III C) factors can account for a discrepancy between receptive and expressive skills (Level III A). As the nature of the discrepant function is assessed and determined, branching to specified juncture points occurs. In III B and C, the notion of clinical uncertainty presents itself. To counter clinical indecision or possible inappropriate nonspeech system adoption, Level IV Motor Speech — Some Contributing Factors and Level V Production — Some Contributing Factors have been included in the decision matrix.

Level IV Motor Speech — Some Contributing Factors. In young or hard-to-test individuals, specifying the presence of a motor speech disorder may be difficult. Consequently, Level IV contains a cluster of factors that are thought to contribute to the diagnosis of neuromotor involvement. These factors include neuromuscular status, eating history, praxic skills, vocal repertoire, and excessive drooling. The practitioner is encouraged to evaluate these factors and use this information for effective decision making.

Level V Production—Some Contributing Factors. Factors included in Level V contribute to an understanding of production deficits. Here a communicator's intelligibility, utterance length, frustration, and use of nonverbal communication forms are studied. As in Level IV, information derived from this level offers evidence for overall decision making.

Level VI Emotional Factors. For some potential nonspeech system candidates, emotional factors exist (e.g., elective mutism) that warrant careful study. The decision matrix attempts to account for this in Level VI Emotional Factors. Careful historical information, including a detailed account for previous therapy, is crucial for appropriate decision making in cases in which the primary etiology is emotionally based.

Level VII Chronological Age Factors. In the decision-making process, chronological age should be considered. However, its influence tends to be one of changing the relative influence or importance of other factors at different ages rather than one of having a solitary effect. Chapman and Miller (1980) suggest that chronological age be used as a standard to compare factors such as development of cognition, comprehension, and production. Although each of the age ranges is listed as a separate factor in the matrix, each leads to the identical outcome. At Level VII A, the practitioner is encouraged to use chronological age as a reminder that the weighing of other factors will vary as a function of age. Accordingly, a 10-year-old nonspeaking child would be viewed differently from a child with similar clinical symptomotology who is 3 years of age. With the 10-year-old, the discrepancy between physical, cognitive, and linguistic functioning and chronological age would tend to exaggerate the lack of expression and influence the election option. With further research, understanding of how age influences decision making and of the predictive ability to identify potential nonspeakers at an earlier age should improve. The earlier we are able to predict that an individual will be nonspeaking, the sooner we can introduce an augmentative communication system that may permit effective communication.

Level VIII Previous Therapy Factors. Previous therapy is a critical juncture in the decision-making process and one that clinicians often overlook in their zeal to effect communicative growth. The factors at this level imply that the practitioner has knowledge of a myriad of speech therapy practices if therapy appropriateness and outcome expectations are to be systematically considered. We prefer that individuals be oral communicators. Consequently, knowing the response to previous speech therapy or allowing time for trial therapy seems obligatory before any decision to elect is made. For this reason, a decision to delay is a frequent outcome at this level.

Level IX Previous Therapy—Some Contributing Factors. Gues, Sailor, and Baer (1978) report that the inability to imitate relates closely with failure in their orally based functional language program. Kent (1974) considers imitation as prerequisite to her language program. We view the ability to imitate as contributing to success in traditional speech therapy programs. The ability is a useful factor in our attempts to decide whether to delay or to elect.

Level X Implementation Factors—Environment. This level is perhaps the most powerful factor in the decision-making process. At this level, the family must decide whether or not to sanction the actual implementation of a recommended nonspeech communication system. Our clinical experience is that for most families, accepting an elect decision is both painful and difficult. Whenever a family is unwilling to implement a system, counseling, in the form of a review and restatement of the factors that led to the decision, is urged. Some individuals have education decisions made by peripherally interested parties. This is often the case with children who are state wards and living in institutional environments. We believe that stronger advocacy at the implementation level would result in more individuals being appropriately placed and making notable progress with augmentative communication systems.

Once the initial decision process has been completed and it has been determined what form of intervention is most appropriate, specific communication goals can be generated. This discussion is prefaced by acknowledging the diverse etiological factors presented by the severely and profoundly handicapped population. Some individuals may present normal or near normal receptive language abilities with severe expressive impairments. Others may demonstrate concurrent receptive as well as expressive language deficits. For this reason, effective communication training strategies are as diverse as the population they are designed to serve. Each individual possesses an array of communication needs which are unique to his or her situation and environment. Communication programs must be designed to fit the needs of each person. Shane (1979) suggests that there are two primary objectives which underlie communication intervention. Naturally, as the individual matures or actually acquires greater skills, more advanced objectives need to be identified, such as (1) to be able to express wants and needs and (2) to be able to describe the here and now. Skill development in these areas not only provides a means of affecting or controlling one's environment (e.g., hunger, thirst, discomfort) but presents a method of communicating current relevant information. Successfully mastering these basic skills can lead to more complex levels of communication and communication devices.

It has been generally recognized (Chapman & Miller, 1980) that the concept of object permanence and means-end relationships are prerequisites to the successful use of communication aids. Initial stages of intervention include consideration of the establishment of skills in Piaget's sensorimotor stage before proceeding.

Shane's communication spiral (1979) depicts stages of communication programming for the speaking or nonspeaking communicator.

As can be seen in Figure 6, the spiral contains five programming levels. The first two are identical for the speaking or nonspeaking communicator since they represent stages each will experience (Shane, 1979). The goals outlined in Levels I and II deal primarily with the refinement of very basic communication skills which enable the nonspeaking person to express wants and needs. At Level II communication performance is typically less dependent on the interpretation of others for the desired item or activity but nonetheless remains dependent on the observational and interpretative skill of caregivers. For example, the nonspeaking person can begin to respond more selectively to questions like "What do you want?" through appropriate motor responses. Instructional efforts during this time are largely devoted to reinforcing responses

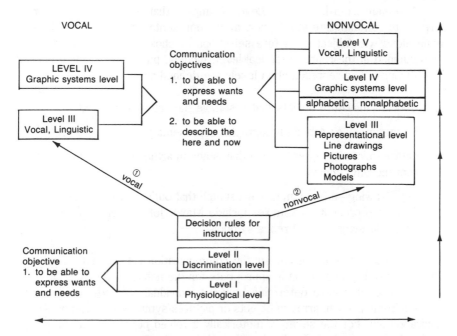

Figure 6. The communication spiral. From Shane (1979, p. 159). Reprinted by permission.

which indicate preference (e.g., toys, food, activities, persons), physiological well-being (e.g., hunger, thirst, pain). Movement from Level II to Level III requires that the communication instructor determine whether speech or augmented techniques training will be implemented. This information is gleaned from the Election Decision Matrix (Shane & Bashir, 1980).

For the speaker upward movement through the spiral does not suggest that augmentative aids like communication boards or alphabet boards are not appropriate to supplement oral communication. Rather, augmentative aids can be utilized to enhance expressive language development as previously suggested (Musselwhite & St. Louis, 1982; Silverman, 1980). Beukelman and Yorkston (1977) concluded from their investigation of the use of alphabet boards with severely dysarthric persons that, when the boards were used to support verbal attempts, intelligibility was markedly improved.

The right side of the spiral is meant to represent the nonvocal, nonspeaking communicator. Upward movement for individuals on this side of the spiral requires training procedures which establish communication aids to augment spoken language as opposed to the support or augmentation of speech attempts. Shane cautions, however, that no two children will progress through the hierarchy in identical ways.

Movement from Level II to Level III implies that the nonspeaking person is ready to communicate at a higher, more representational level. This is commonly done with object or picture selections or choices. Four sublevels have been outlined in the representational level: models, photographs, pictures, and line drawings. The representation levels are defined as follows:

1. Models—miniature objects that resemble the actual object.

2. Photographs—an actual photographic representation of a real object.

3. Picture—pictorial representation that is not an actual photograph of an object from the environment.

4. Line Drawing—a two-dimensional sketch that outlines the parameter of the object it represents. Examples include Mayer-Johnson line drawings, Picsyms, Blissymbols, and rebus symbols.

It then becomes important for the communication instructor to determine which level of representation is appropriate for the nonspeaking student.

The next step is to determine how the individual can most easily select intended items from an array of objects or pictures/symbols arranged on a communication aid. For the severely motorically involved person it may be necessary to design a method of indication since direct selection is not always a viable alternative. Single switches can be used to control various electronic communication aids and displays. Appendix E contains only a limited sample of the switches constructed for the severely physically involved person. These switches attempt to capitalize on any consistent motor response the individual can produce. When paired with a single switch, scanning and encoding communication systems can become powerful choice selection indicators. Nonelectronic methods or alternative indication might include mouth sticks and headsticks.

Movement to Level IV, the graphics system level, indicates that the student has demonstrated skills which would indicate development of a system accommodating the combination of symbols or pictures to represent entire thoughts or ideas. Graphic systems are divided into two categories: nonalphabetic and alphabetic symbols. Nonalphabetic symbols can represent one or more words or ideas (e.g., Picsyms, rebus, or Blissymbols). Notice in Figure 7 how four entirely different symbol sets can be used to construct the same message.

Alphabetic symbols or traditional orthography is the most desired and recognized form of representation. It presents some advantages and disadvantages in terms of the persons who can successfully use it as a foundation for communication. The most obvious advantage, of course, is the potential it holds for utilizing microcomputer systems which will enable the nonspeaking person, with special modifications, to participate in traditional educational and vocational settings. Many of the communication aids presently available use standard orthographic representation in their displays. The apparent disadvantage is that the user must possess the skills necessary to interpret and utilize this form of representation in order to read and write. For the physically handicapped as well as the cognitively low-functioning individual who will never read or write, the absence of these skills presents barriers to successful use of many electronic communication aids. Table 3 outlines the advantages and disadvantages of alphabetic and nonalphabetic systems.

The final level represented in the communication spiral is the vocal linguistic level. Intervention at this level may occur for a variety of reasons. Misdiagnosis or change in the status of expressive language abilities are among the possible reasons for intervention at this level. In summary, it is up to the communication instructor to strategically plan the horizontal or vertical movement through the spiral. The following guidelines are offered to further assist the decision-making process (Shane, 1979).

These are suggestions to help communication instructors get started in working with those persons whose communication has been characterized by caregiver interpretation of behavior rather than by voluntary expression of wants and needs. These guidelines have been particularly useful at Level II for teaching a student that this behavior (e.g., point or eye gaze) can affect his or her

Friend   I/Me   to go, to leave   restaurant

i+ ♡T   ⌐T   ↑< |o⌐|

my   friend (-s, -'s, -ly)   I I   go (-ing, -s)   diningroom (-s, -'s)

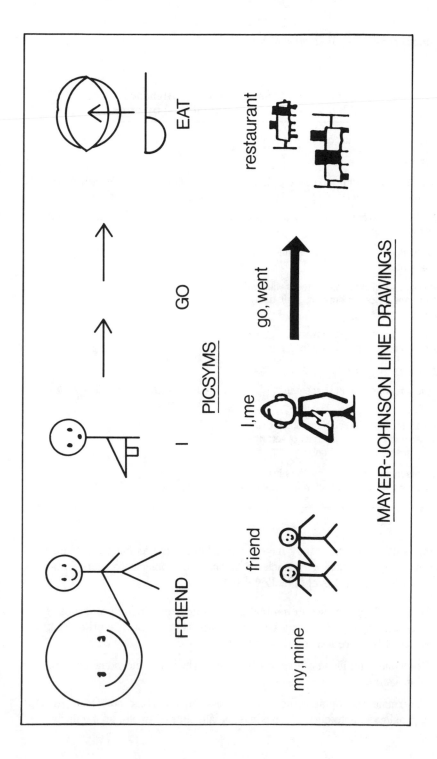

Figure 7. Nonalphabetic symbol symbols.

TABLE 3
Advantages and Disadvantages of Alphabetic
and Nonalphabetic Representational Systems

Advantages	Disadvantages
Nonalphabetic	
1. Can be used with cognitively low-functioning individuals	1. Availability of electronic aids is limited
2. Can be used to construct complex messages or ideas	2. Not as widely accepted as alphabetic representation
3. Easily used to initiate communication programming	
4. Aids can be easily constructed by family members or other support staff using these symbols	
5. Can be used as precursor to more sophisticated techniques and aids	
Alphabetic	
1. Widely recognized and accepted	1. Requires high-level cognitive skills (e.g., reading, writing, etc.)
2. Electronic systems can be modified to increase participation in a variety of settings (e.g., work, home, school)	
3. Representational system commonly used in electronic communication devices	

environment. In addition, they have been helpful in overcoming the often difficult yet significant training obstacle of moving from objects to representations of objects (i.e., from Level II to Level III).

1. Select high-preference items that have natural reinforcing properties (e.g., a record player that provides musical entertainment or a favorite drink) or, at Level III, a representation of those items.

2. Determine the highest level on the spiral where the individual can process information.

3. Determine the optimal mode of expression (vocal or nonvocal). Accept approximations to correct response initially. For example, an intelligible yet

misarticulated utterance or a grossly accurate but not precise pointing response can be used as an indication.

4. Place the student before the object or representation of object.

5. Require a manding response (i.e., must touch, point to, pick up, or verbally label the high-preference item). By a correct response, the individual specifies his or her reinforcement and is allowed to interact with the object for a given period of time.

6. Allow for spontaneous expression of wants and needs. Once a student responds to a command, such as "What do you want?" or "Point to the cup," consider developing strategies that will allow spontaneous expression.

7. Begin vertical and horizontal movement through the spiral.

Selection and Implementation of an Augmentative Communication Aid

Augmentative communication aids can have a significant impact on all aspects of the nonspeaking person's life. While the potential remains for these aids to impact educational and vocational opportunities, appropriate steps must be taken to ensure that they are selected and implemented appropriately. These decisions must be made carefully because of the effects produced in the life of the handicapped individual and those with whom they interact.

The Interdisciplinary Model

Because of the enormity of the physical, intellectual, and linguistic problems presented by the nonspeaking population, the input of a number of professionals is required in order to make adequate decisions. The common denominator in this team is an understanding of the communicative needs of the population as a whole and an appreciation of available programs and technique options. Having such an orientation, each professional can then contribute his or her specialized expertise (Cohen & Shane, 1982). The speech and language pathologist can play a primary role in the coordination and implementation of services for the nonspeaking person (ASHA, 1980). This opinion originates from the experience of speech and language pathologists in the assessment of motor speech capability and overall communication needs (Cohen & Shane, 1982). Cohen and Shane (1982) present a list of "ideal" members or professionals whose input may provide crucial direction in meeting the needs of the nonspeaking person. The members of this team are listed in Table 4.

TABLE 4
Components of Ideal Nonspeech Evaluation and Service Delivery Team
for Potential User of Aided and/or Unaided Communication Technique

1. Advocate	8. Education
2. Follow-through coordinator	9. Medicine
3. Fabrication specialist	10. Occupational therapy
4. Fitting specialist (interface and electronic aid aspect)	11. Parent/caregiver
	12. Physical therapy
5. Audiology	13. Psychology
6. Biomedical engineering	14. Social service
7. Competent manual signer	15. Speech-language pathology

Source: Cohen and Shane (1982, p. 876).

An examination of Table 4 reveals that fewer specialists are generally involved when the decision to augment communication is an unaided technique since the personnel involved in selling, developing, and fitting an aided system are not involved. Furthermore, due to the complex nature of motor problems commonly experienced by nonspeaking clients, a host of medical personnel might be involved at some level in the assessment and program planning. After initial assessment procedures are completed, follow-up services which include the education and training of the system user and all other related persons or professionals should be given full attention. Table 5 contains a list of these professionals and their areas of expertise on such a team (Yorkston & Karlan, 1986).

The program plan which results from such an assessment is a product of the age, environment (e.g., school, work, home), and communicative needs of the nonspeaking person. Since communication development is an ongoing process, continued reevaluation is needed in order to expand the communication system and meet changing needs (Shane & Yoder, 1981).

Shane & Yoder (1981) report that, for the school-age child, program progress and communication aid construction can be monitored through the IEP format of quarterly and annual reviews. These authors further suggest the incorporation of the following guidelines in communication program development:

1. Has the user's current level of performance with regard to linguistic, cognitive, and motor capabilities been documented?

2. Is the system functional?

3. Is it preparatory in nature?

TABLE 5
Areas of Expertise on an Augmentative Communication Team

Speech-Language Pathology
    Normal and disordered communication
    Language development and disorders in normal and disordered populations
    Motor speech disorders
    Alternative and augmentative approaches
Medicine
    Management of therapeutic programs
    Natural course of the disorder
    Medical intervention
    Management of medication regimes
Physical Therapy
    Mobility aids
    Motor control and motor learning
    Positioning to maximizing functioning
    Maintenance of strength and range of motion
    Physical conditioning to increase flexibility, balance, and coordination
Occupational Therapy
    Activities of daily living
    Positioning to maximize function
    Adaptive equipment
Engineering
    Application and modification of existing electronic or mechanical aids and devices
Computer Technology
    Modification of existing software program
    Development of programs to meet existing needs
    Evaluation of software program for potential use by clients
Education
    Development and sequencing of appropriate social and academic experiences
    Development of cognitive/conceptual objectives
    Assessment of sociocommunicative functioning
    Development of an appropriate vocational curriculum
Social Services
    Evaluation of total living situation
Vocational Counseling
    Assessment of vocational potential
    Identification of vocational goals
Other Areas of Consultation
    Audiology
    Ophthamology
    Orthopedics
    Neurology
    Rehabilitation nursing
    Prosthetic

Source: Yorkston and Karlan (1986).

4. Is it individualized?

5. Does it provide for interactions with handicapped peers and other persons?

6. Does it allow for at least partial participation in a wide variety of instructional arrangements (e.g., one-to-one, group, and so forth)?

7. Are individual adaptations accomplished which maximize participation?

8. Can it accommodate a variety of instructional arrangements (e.g., one-to-one, group, and so forth)?

9. Are there strategies developed for continuous assessment and documentation of outcomes?

10. Are the teaching techniques used providing salient instruction?

11. Is it free of "dead time"?

12. Does it allow for the coordination of instruction and related services?

13. Can daily lesson plans be written for its implementation?

14. Is it consistent with the user's effective and sensory characteristics?

Although these guidelines were originally formulated for the development of IEP school programs, they can provide assistance for the delineation of communication programs for other settings as well.

Since communication occurs throughout the day in multiple settings, training should be emphasized at varying times in each setting. Furthermore, parents, spouse, friends, and others should be involved in the training process. Designing programs which invite the participation of significant communication partners can only strengthen the transition of communication skills across settings, persons, and time. Strategies should be developed which encourage this. Environmental inventories can provide information to ensure that communication programming maintains its relevancy and functionality for the user. From this very specific approach, communication goals can be ascertained. Typical considerations include:

1. What are the response routines required in that setting?
2. Is the user required to initiate messages?
3. Is the user predominantly the message receiver?

These questions need to be considered for each new person, and in each new setting the questions must be asked again. Programming, like evaluation, is an ongoing process. The overall goal, however, is the development of effective interaction. It is likely that the communication/interaction system will consist of several communication techniques to be used at different times, depending upon which is most functional at a given time, with a given audience, and under given circumstances (Harris & Vanderheiden, 1980a).

System Design

Designing a communication system which will provide opportunities for the user to communicate effectively is a primary concern. In Table 6 Vanderheiden and Lloyd (1986) present a comprehensive checklist of the requirements of an overall multitechnique strategy. The multitechnique strategy system encourages the use of a collection of techniques, aids, and strategies (some aided, some unaided) that the individual uses interchangeably. System selection (electronic or non-electronic), training the user to communicate successfully with the aid as well as other involved communication partners, and selection of an appropriate symbol system are all prerequisites to the successful implementation of a communication aid. However, the prescription of an aid which does not appropriately meet the needs of the user or communication interactants can restrict rather than enhance communication attempts. A number of factors must be taken into consideration. One of the first considerations is that the system is age appropriate. Furthermore, it must serve present communication needs as well as potential future needs. If a designated aid serves the child's needs at home, can the utility of the aid be expanded to encompass those demands at school? These types of educational and environmental determinations can have monumental effects on effective communication aid use in the present and future.

Parent/guardian/caregiver preferences or cooperation using the aid will effectively enhance or diminish the ability to develop skills to support the use of an aid. Since it is the parent/guardian/caregiver who assumes the major responsibility for satisfying daily living needs and following through with established communication goals, it is only reasonable to suggest that during the selection process these persons should be given priority in final selection decisions. Potential communication partners need to feel confident in their ability to communicate with the nonspeaking person using the prescribed aid. Communication is only reinforcing when the exchange of information is successful and the message successfully transmitted. If the selected aid is not a useful tool during these exchanges of information, it is highly probable that the user and his or her partner will use alternative modes of communication. This becomes a problem most often when the communication partner does not approve of the selected aid. Therefore, if aid selection proceeds with client and caregiver preferences in mind, the probability that the aid will be incorporated is significantly

TABLE 6
Requirements of an Overall MTS Communication System: A Checklist

Provides full range of communicative functions:
  Communication of basic needs
  Conversation
  Writing (and messaging?)
  Computer access (electronic communication, learning, and information systems)

Is compatible with:
  Seating system and *all* other positions
  Mobility
  Environmental controls
  Other devices, teaching approaches, etc., in the environment

Does not restrict communication partners:
  Totally obvious yes/no for strangers (from 3–5 feet away – the closest they some-
  times come)
  Usable/understandable with strangers and those not familiar with special techniques
  or symbols
  Promotes face-to-face communication
  Usable with peers/community
  Usable with groups

Does not restrict communication environments/physical positions:
  Is always with the person (always working)
  Functions in noisy environments
  Withstands physically hostile environments (sandbox, beach, travel, classroom)

Does not restrict communication topic or scope:
  Any topic, word, idea expressible
  Open vocabulary
  User-definable vocabulary

enhanced. Along the same continuum is the question of functionality. As previously determined, a communication aid must meet a variety of needs in a variety of settings. The physically handicapped college student, for example, may need a device with speech output capabilities for answering and asking questions in class and conversation. Upon returning home each evening the system may serve a variety of other functions. In addition to a simple voice output device this student needs a tool to assist him or her in completing assignments, turning on and off appliances, and using the phone. In this case system design must account for all these needs and, above all, provide a functional means of accomplishing each of these tasks. Of course, not all nonspeaking persons present needs as complex as this. For some persons a nonelectronic communication aid

TABLE 6. Continued

Is effective:
Maximum possible rate (for both Quicktalk and Exactalk)
Very quick method for key message (phatic, emergency, control)(Quicktalk)
Yes/no communicable from a distance
Basic needs communication from a distance (at least alerting)
Ability to interrupt and fight off interruptions
Ability to control message (e.g., finish it and not be "interpreted")
Ability to overlay emphasis or emotion on top of message
Low fatigue
Special superefficient techniques for those close to individual

Fosters and allows growth:
Appropriate to individual's current skills
Allows vocabulary, topic, grammar, function growth
New vocabulary, aspects easily learned

Is accepted and motivates user and significant others
Individual
Family
Peers/friends
Education or employment environment

Is affordable
Purchase
Maintenance
Need for assistant

Source: Vanderheiden and Lloyd (1986).

may more appropriately meet their needs. Nonetheless it does serve to exemplify a very important consideration in system design—functionality. This leads to yet another consideration. A communication system must enable the user to move it from place to place. The nonambulatory person can use a wheelchair laptray for attaching an aid. Communication aids recommended for the ambulatory nonspeaking person are typically smaller and feature modifications which enhance portability, such as shoulder straps. If an aid is too large and cumbersome to allow it to be easily transported, it will probably not be used. Once again this can be addressed most appropriately by determining where and how the aid is to be used. Table 7 (Vanderheiden & Lloyd, 1986) presents a com-

TABLE 7
Important Functional Dimensions of Individual Techniques or Approaches*

Dimension	Definition	Importance/Impact
Functionality/ability to meet needs		
Openness	Ability to express any thought	Open topic access Allows individual to advance on own
Speed	Rate of communication	More effective Easier for younger and retarded
Assertability	Ability to interrupt; resist interruptions; and control conversation	More effective Prevents frustration, shutdown
Display permanence	Permanence of the presentation or display (temporary dynamic, temporary static, displayed, printed)	Meets writing needs Provides time to decipher Access to other words through cues Rate—don't need to wait for message receiver Feedback for growth, learning
Projection	Ability to communicate at a distance	Communicate to/with groups Communicate at a distance
Correctibility	Ability to unambiguously repair or correct utterances	Clarity True representation Learning Motivation Motivating
Expandability	Ability to expand function, use, or vocabulary by user, by others	Expand topics Allows growth
Availability/usability		
Portability	Ability to conveniently stay with the person at all times	Can go with user
Position independence	Ability to be used in any and all positions (wheelchair, couch, standing, lying down)	Increases availability Use with people in certain environments (e.g., home)
Independence	Lack of need for an assistant or interpreter	Effectiveness Motivating Lower cost to use
Intelligibility/obviousness	Ability of technique to be understood by strangers	More potential communication partners, strangers Ease of learning

*Some of these apply to the symbol portion of a technique, some to the transmission mode, some to both.

TABLE 7. Continued

Dimension	Definition	Importance/Impact
Appropriateness	Appropriate to individual's current and future abilities (physical, cognitive, language)	For effectiveness For growth
Durability	Ruggedness, indestructibility, reliability	Available for use (not broken) Can go with user to more places
Total cost	Cost of purchase, maintenance, training, and assistants or aides required for use	Cost

Acceptability/compatibility with the environment

Cosmesis	Appearance, attractiveness	Acceptability Communication partners (e.g., removal in public)
Material/practice compatibility	Compatibility of technique with materials and practices of educational or employment settings	Usability at school or job Acceptability to teachers, employers
Similarity	Similarity to communication system of peers and community	More communication partners Models for the user More acceptable
Training required	Amount of training required of user, therapists, others	Learnability when resources are limited Cost overall
Adaptability	Ability to be customized to individual's needs, abilities, and constraints	Adapt to user's other aids Vocabulary Fine-tune for speed, function
Computer compatibility	Ability to implement the technique or symbols on standard computers	Low-cost writing system Computer-aided teaching Lower cost implementation
Interdevice compatibility	Ability to use the approach/technique with other standard devices in the environment	Access to electronic communication, learning, or information systems in environment

Source: Vanderheiden and Lloyd (1986).

pilation of important functional dimensions of individual techniques or approaches and lists some of the considerations used in selecting an input or output system.

Vocabulary Selection

Vocabulary selection is crucial to successful implementation of electronic or nonelectronic aids. Although the vocabulary selected for the cognitively low-functioning client will not be as complex, the means by which this selection occurs is typical to any client.

Selection will be influenced by personal experiences, cognitive abilities, and linguistic history. High-preference items possessing naturally reinforcing properties (e.g., favorite activities, persons, or items) should be incorporated. Vocabulary representing feelings (e.g., humor, frustration, anger, happiness) should also be available.

Generally items or concepts should be chosen which are easily demonstrated with any symbol system, alphabetic or nonalphabetic. The final selection would then include those items, concepts, and ideas which are useful to the communicator and the communication partner in their interactions. Keeping a daily log of activities and interests can provide important insight for vocabulary selection.

Case Examples

This section includes a brief description of several individual cases. The following cases include an adult, a teenager, and a child. The age, etiology, history, and prescribed communication approach will be described.

Case 1. Michael

Onset: Age 2
Approach: Environmentally specific minicommunication boards
Etiology: Profound brain injury
Age: 9

History:

Michael was the product of profound brain injury suffered as a result of nearly drowning at the age of 2. Michael experienced limited functional expressive communication. With the exception of a few context-specific situations, communication was comprised of unintelligible vocalizations. Furthermore, Michael was nonambulatory and was dependent on primary caregivers for transportation, feeding, and daily care. Hypertonic muscle tone was observed to increase with intention.

Evaluation:

During the evaluation Michael did not demonstrate response modes (e.g., visual tracking and attending skills), which would support the development of a sophisticated communication system as suggested by Level I of the decision matrix (see Figure 5). Therefore, the decision was made to delay until appropriate training had been undertaken and Michael developed skills which would support development of an augmentative communication system.

Recommendations:

Recommendations included establishing visual attention and tracking skills as well as developing responses to choice presentations of objects using eye gaze, a method of indication. Adaptive toys were recommended to increase active stimulation and environmental interaction. His parents were also urged to keep encouraging Michael to express preferences for objects and activities by whatever means possible (vocalizations, etc.). A re-evaluation was then scheduled in 3 months.

Case 2. Bill

Onset: Congenital
Approach: Prentke Romich Light Talker
Etiology: Cerebral palsy
Age: 15

History:

Bill is a 15-year-old young man with a moderately severe athetoid type of cerebral palsy. Bill was referred to the clinic by school staff and parents. Speech was highly unintelligible to all but familiar communication interactants. School work was completed on a microcomputer system with the assistance of special education aid. Due to the nature of Bill's motor involvement, he could activate keys most accurately using his toes. Bill was nonambulatory, but he independently transported himself from place to place with a walker constructed by his father. Using the walker, he participated in activities at school like kickball. Although he demonstrated precise lower-extremity control, his most consistent and controlled movement was observed to be his head control. A number of issues needed to be addressed in order to effectively implement a communication aid:

1. The aid must remain portable to allow transportation on his walker or an electric wheelchair.
2. The aid must possess speech output capability to supplement Bill's unintelligible communication attempts.
3. Mounting an aid at the foot of Bill's walker or wheelchair created transporting problems, so another method of indication was investigated.
4. The aid must support Bill's participation in a normal classroom setting by permitting him to successfully and efficiently complete classroom assignments.

Evaluation:
      In addition to the needs outlined above, Bill presented a number of other skills which led to the final system selection. According to the decision matrix, the decision to implement an augmentative communication system was made in the following way:
      Level I Cognitive Factors. Bill easily met this criteria of stage V sensorimotor intelligence. Continue to Level II.
      Level II Oral Reflex Factors. No persistent oral reflex factors present. Continue to Level III.
      Level III Language and Motor Speech Production Factors. The discrepancy in Bill's receptive and expressive language was based predominantly on a motor speech disorder. Go to Level V.
      Level V Production. Bill's speech was unintelligible except to family or familiar communication partners, which meant that it was necessary to supplement his speech with gross pointing or gestures. Once again an affirmative response at this level suggests movement to Level VII.
      Level VII Chronological Age Factors. Bill's chronological age was 15. Go to Level VIIIA.
      Level VIIIA. Due to the extensive motor involvement associated with Bill's cerebral palsy, it was determined that therapy had appropriately been withheld, which led to the final decision to implement an augmentative communication aid at Level X.

Recommendations:
      The Prentke Romich Light Talker was the system of choice. Bill demonstrated excellent head control, which could be used as a control site. The Light

Talker could then be mounted to his wheelchair or walker and contains an independent energy supply, thereby contributing to its portability. Furthermore, this device has speech output and can independently store information for completion of school assignments or can be interfaced with a microcomputer system for standard computer operation and the use of standard software.

Case 3. Glen

Onset: Congenital
Approach: Communication book, sign language, and Sharp Memowriter
Etiology: Hearing impairment, mild retardation, spastic cerebral palsy
Age: 37

History:
   Glen is a 37-year-old man with a severe to profound sensorineural hearing loss. He lived at home with his parents before moving into a group residential setting. Although Glen demonstrated a mild form of mental retardation, he was able to read and write on approximately a fifth-grade level. Glen's communication problems involved communicating with persons who did not know sign language in the community. He was successfully placed in a vocational position entering simple line text into a word processor. This meant that he came in contact with a variety of individuals who were not and were never going to become signing communicators. Furthermore, since Glen was nonspeaking and ambulatory, an appropriate system recommendation weighed heavily on portability factors.

Evaluation:
   Glen's recommendations were based on a process very similar to that of Bill. However, Glen's inability to communicate effectively with speech was not due primarily to a motor speech problem but to his hearing impairment. All other factors were the same, which led to the implementation of an augmentative communication aid but with a different design.

Recommendation:
   Glen was reluctant to use a communication aid when the opportunity to sign presented itself. He therefore needed a system which could most easily supplement these skills. Speech output was not an important factor to Glen or the environment he lived in due to his hearing impairment. From the beginning Glen made it quite clear that he would not carry or use a device that was larger

then he felt it should be. His ability to read and write lent nicely to the recommendation of the Sharp Memowriter, a portable typewriter which weighs less
than one pound. It has the capacity to store frequently used words and phrases,
thus contributing to communication enhancement. Glen was able to successfully
communicate with those in his work setting and in the community, and the Sharp
Memowriter was small enough to be carried in a small bag with a shoulder strap.
A small communication board was constructed to provide a backup system should
the Memowriter malfunction. In addition, because many of Glen's roommates
in his residential setting did not read, the communication board was constructed
with pictographic symbols to allow Glen to communicate with them as well.

Conclusion

Today's technology is helping improve the chances of the nonspeaking physically handicapped person's ability to effectively participate in society. Microcomputer systems have made it possible to perform educational and vocational tasks,
speech synthesizers have given the nonspeaking a voice, and environmental
controls have provided a more independent way of meeting daily needs and
controlling household utilities. However, communication for the nonspeaking
individual still remains a slow, arduous task and oftentimes quite impersonal.
The systems of tomorrow will need to potentially increase the rate of communication as well as become more personalized. This appears to be happening
with the advent of high-quality speech synthesizers which are user-definable. In
other words, the user can design a voice which will more readily duplicate his
or her own voice or any desired. These barriers must be overcome if the nonspeaking population is to have a role as productive members of our society. As
Daniel Webster noted, "If my possessions were taken from me with one exception, I would choose to keep the power of communication, for by it I would
soon regain all the rest."

Appendices

Appendix A
Informational Resources

Directories for Microcomputer Software

The Handicapped Source
101 Rt. 46 East
Pine Brook, NJ 07058
(free catalogue)

*Trace Center Software/Hardware
    Registry*
University of Wisconsin – Madison
S151 Waisman Center
1500 Highland Avenue
Madison, WI 53706

*Compilation of Clinical Software for
    Aphasia Rehabilitation and
    Cognitive Retraining*
Clinical Software Resources
2850 Windmere
Birmingham, MI 48008
($69.95)

Schneier Communication Unit
Cerebral Palsy Center
1603 Court Street
Syracuse, NY 13208
(SCU software list: preschool
    software companies)

Software Registry – Third Edition
CUSH
James Fitch, Editor
Department of Speech Pathology
    and Audiology
University of South Alabama
Mobile, AL 36688
(Software in the areas of
    communication disorders)

*Source Listing for Microcomputer
    Software for Special Education*
LINC Resources, Incorporated
1875 Morse Road, Suite 225
Columbus, OH 43229
(also available from LINC, Special
    Ware Director, 1983)

*The 1984 Educational Software
    Preview Guide*
Center for Learning Technologies
Cultural Education Center
Room 9A47
Albany, NY 12230

*Handbook of Microcomputer
    Applications in Communication
    Disorders*
A. Schwartz, Editor
San Diego, CA: College Hill Press
(Contains information on clinical and
    administrative software)

*Microcomputer Resource Book for
    Special Education*
D. Hagen
Reston Publishing Company
(Contains information on clinical and
    administrative software)

Communication Enhancement Clinic
The Children's Hospital
300 Longwood Avenue
Boston, MA 02115
(Software listing)

Additional Sources for Software/Hardware Information

*International Software Registry of
  Programs Written or Adapted for
  Individuals*
Trace Research and Development
  Center
S151 Waisman Center
1500 Highland Avenue
Madison, WI 53705
($25.00)

Institute on Technology
Fegan 9
300 Longwood Avenue
Boston, MA 02115

Link and Go
2030 Irving Park Boulevard
Chicago, IL 60618

Closing the Gap
P. O. Box 68
Henderson, MN 56044
(newspaper dealing with technology
  for handicapped children and
  adults)

*Computer Users in Speech and
  Hearing* (CUSH)
Department of Speech Pathology
  and Audiology
University of South Alabama
Mobile, AL 36688
(Newsletter dealing with computer
  application in communication
  disorders)

Communication Outlook
Artificial Language Laboratory
Computer Science Department
Michigan State University
East Lansing, MI 48824
(Newsletter on augmentative
  communication)

*Journal of Special Educational
  Technology*
Exceptional Child Center
Utah State University
Logan, UT 84322

*Bulletin on Science and Technology
  for the Handicapped*
AAAS
1515 Massachusetts Avenue, NW
Washington, DC 20005

Computer-Disability News
National Easter Seal Society
2023 West Ogdon Avenue
Chilcago, IL 60612
(Newsletter focusing on computers
  for disabled individuals)

The Exceptional Parent
605 Commonwealth Avenue
Boston, MA 02215
(A magazine for parents of
  handicapped children)

Appendix B
Distributors

Adaptive Communication Systems, Inc.
Box 12440, Pittsburgh, PA 15231
(412) 264-2288

Adaptive Peripherals
4529 Bagley Avenue N., Seattle, WA 98103
(206) 633-2610

Apple Computer, Inc.
20525 Mariani Drive, Cupertino, CA 95014
(408) 996-1010

Cacti Computer Services
130 9th Street, S.W., Portage La Prairie, Manitoba, R1N 2N4
(204)857-8675
Note: Import fees significantly increase the cost of small orders.

Canon USA, Inc.
One Canon Plaza, Lake Success, NY 11043
(516) 488-6700

Charles Ladd
Star Route 1, Box 110, Bristol, NH 03222

Digital Equipment Corporation
Maynard, MA 01754
(617) 987-5111

Communication Enhancement Clinic
Children's Hospital
300 Longwood Avenue, Boston, MA 02115
(617) 735-6466

Don Johnston Developmental Equipment
981 Winnetka Terrace, Lake Zurich, IL 60047
(312) 438-3476

Dunamis, Inc.
2856 Buford Highway, Duluth GA 30136
(404) 476-4934

Epson America
3415 Kashiwa Street, Torrance, CA 90505
(213) 539-9140

Handicapped Children's Technological Services
P.O. Box 7, Foster, RI 02825
(401) 397-7666

Institute on Technology
Fegan 9, 300 Longwood Avenue, Boston, MA 02115
(617) 735-7870

Intex Micro Systems Corporation
725 South Adams Road, Birmingham, MI 48011
(313) 540-7601

Jostens Learning Systems/Borg Warner
600 West University Drive, Arlington Heights, IL 60004
(800) 323-7577

Koala Technologies, Inc.
3100 Patrick Henry Drive, Santa Clara, CA 95050
(408) 986-8866

Marbel Systems
P.O. Box 750, Exeter, NH 03833
(603) 778-7768

MCE, Inc.
157 South Kalamazoo Mall, Suite
  250, Kalamazoo, MI 49007
(800) 421-4157

Prentke Romich Company
1022 Heyl Road, Wooster, OH
  44691
(216) 262-1984

Santech Ltd.
P.O. Box 231, Brooklyn Park, South
  Australia 5032

Steven Kanor, Inc.
8 Main Street, Hastings-on-Hudson,
  NY 10706
(914) 478-0960

Street Electronics Corporation
1140 Mark Avenue, Carpenteria,
  CA 93013
(805) 684-4593

Sweet Micro Systems
50 Freeway Drive, Cranston, RI
  02920
(401) 461-0530

Tash
70 Gibson Drive, Unit 1, Markham,
  Ontario, L3R 2Z4
(416) 475-2212
Note: Import fees significantly
  increase the cost of small orders.

Unicorn Engineering Company
6201 Harwood Avenue, Oakland,
  CA 94618
(415) 428-1626

Votrax, Inc.
1394 Rankin, Troy, MI 48083-4074
(313) 588-2050

Words +, Inc.
1125 Stewart Court, Suite D.,
  Sunnyvale, CA 94086
(408) 730-9588

Zygo Industries, Inc.
P.O. Box 1008, Portland, OR
  97207-1008
(503) 297-1724

Appendix C
Suggested Readings

Population Characteristics

Darley, F. L., Aronson, A. E., & Brown, M. D. (1975). *Motor speech disorders.* Philadelphia: W. B. Saunders Co.

Silverman, F. (1980). *Communication for the speechless.* Englewood Cliffs, NJ: Prentice-Hall.

Overview of Terminology and Historical Perspective

Bonvillian, J. D., & Nelson, K. E. (1976). Sign language acquisition in a mute autistic boy. *Journal of Speech and Hearing Disorders, 41,* 339–347.

Carrier, J. K., Jr. (1976). Application of non-speech language system with the severely language handicapped. In L. L. Lloyd (Ed.), *Communication assessment and intervention strategies* (pp. 523–547). Austin, TX: PRO-ED.

Fristoe, M., & Lloyd, L. L. (1978). A survey of the use of non-speech systems with the severely communication impaired. *Mental Retardation, 16,* 99–103.

Kiernan, C. (1973). Alternatives to speech: A review of research on manual and other alternative forms of communication with the mentally handicapped. *British Journal of Mental Subnormality, 23,* 6–28.

Lloyd, L. L., & Karlan, G. A. (1984). Non-speech communication symbols and systems: Where have we been and where are we going? *Journal of Mental Deficiency Research, 28,* 3–9.

McDonald, E. T., & Schultz, A. R. (1973). Communications boards for cerebral-palsied children. *Journal of Speech and Hearing Disorders, 38,* 73–88.

Vicker, B. (Ed.). (1974). *Non-oral communication system project 1964/73.* Iowa City: Campus Stores.

Evaluation/Election/Selection

Chapman, R., & Miller, J. F. (1980). Analyzing language and communication in the child. In R. L. Schiefelbusch (Ed.), *Nonspeech language and communication: Analysis and intervention* (pp. 159–196). Austin, TX: PRO-ED.

Coleman, C. L., Cook, A. M., & Myers, L. S. (1980). Assessing non-oral clients for assistive communication devices. *Journal of Speech and Hearing Disorders, 45,* 515–526.

Ferrier, L. J., & Shane, H. C. (1983). A description of a non-speaking population under consideration for augmentative communication systems. In J. Hogg & P. J. Mittler (Eds.), *Advances in mental handicap research: Vol. 2* (pp. 95–137). Chichester, NY: John Wiley & Sons.

Shane, H. C. (1980). Approaches to assessing the communication of non-oral persons. In R. L. Schiefelbusch (Ed.), *Nonspeech language and communication: Analysis and intervention* (pp. 155–179). Austin, TX: PRO-ED.

Shane, H. C., & Bashir, A. S. (1980). Election criteria for the adoption of an augmentative communication system: Preliminary considerations. *Journal of Speech and Hearing Disorders, 45,* 408–414.

Appendix D
Intervention

Blackstone, S. W., & Cassat-James, E. L. (1984, October). *Communication competence in communication aid users and their partners.* Paper presented at the Third International Conference on augmentative and alternative communication, Boston.

Clarke, C. R., & Woodcock, R. W. (1976). Graphic systems of communications. In L. L. Lloyd (Ed.), *Communication assessment and intervention strategies* (pp. 549–606). Austin, TX: PRO-ED.

Ferrier, L. J., & Shane, H. C. (1981). Communication skills. In J. Umbreit & Cardullias (Eds.), *Educating the severely physically handicapped: Curriculum adaptations.* Columbus, OH: Special Press.

Goodenough-Trepagnier, C., & Prather, P. (1981). Communication systems for the nonvocal based on frequent phoneme sequences. *Journal of Speech and Hearing Research, 24,* 322–329.

Harris, D., & Vanderheiden, G. C. (1980). Augmentative communication techniques. In G. C. Vanderheiden & K. Grilley (Eds.), *Non-vocal communication techniques and aids for the severely physically handicapped.* Austin, TX: PRO-ED.

Musselwhite, C. R., & St. Louis, K. W. (1982). *Communication programming for the severely handicapped* (pp. 158–185). San Diego: College Hill Press.

Shane, H. C. (1979). Approaches to communication training with people who are severely handicapped. In R. York & G. Edgar (Eds.), *Teaching the severely handicapped: Vol. IV.* Columbus, OH: Special Press.

Technological Approaches to Augmentative Communication

Kraat, A., & Sitver-Kogut, M. (1984). *Features of commercially available communication aids.* Prentke Romich Co., 1022 Heyl Road, Wooster, OH.

Traynor, C. D., & Beukelman, D. R. (1984). Non-vocal communication augmentation using microcomputers. *Exceptional Education Quarterly, 4,* 90–103.

Vanderheiden, G. C. (1980). Technology needs of individuals with communication impairments. *Seminar in Speech and Language, 5,* 59–67.

Vocabulary Selection

Blau, A. F. (1983). Vocabulary selection in augmentative communication: Where do we begin? In H. Winitz (Ed.), *Treating language disorders: For clinicians, by clinicians.* Austin, TX: PRO-ED.

Carlson, F. (1981). A format for selecting vocabulary for the non-speaking child. *Language, Speech, and Hearing Services in Schools, 12,* 240–248.

Karlan, G. R., & Lloyd, L. L. (1983). Consideration in the planning of communication intervention: Selecting a lexicon. *TASH Journal, 8.*

Appendix E
Control Interfaces

Acoustic Pickup
Unit for transforming sound to electrical pulses for controlling apparatus in the linguadue range. The position of the individual relative to the microphone is not critical.

Air Cushion Chin Switch
Switch is operated by touching the soft air bellows with the chin. The air bellows and chest plate are drool-proof and washable.

Air Cushion Pneumatic Switch
Sensitive air bellows are activated by slight touch of any body part. Upon activation, a low-pressure air pulse is sent through the tubing to a remote pressure switch. It can be used in moist areas and can be washed since the control portion and PVC tubing are non-electric.

Arm Slot Control
Switches are activated when the user places an arm on one of the four paddles. The paddles are arranged in an arc with barriers between each one to prevent the arm from sliding off the paddle.

Arm Slot Control (five micro switches)
Permits directional scanning and can be activated by gross arm, hand, or foot movement. Appropriate for operation of communication aids.

Brow Wrinkle Switch
This lightweight switch uses small movements of the brow or wrist for activation. Appropriate for row-column and linear scanning of communication aids.

Button Switch
Light pressure on either button will activate switch. Usually used with fingers, elbows, feet, or a headstick.

Chin Switch
The switch is activated by using the chin. It incorporates rocking level switches that are mounted on a chest plate that is worn by the user. Adjustable straps and a ball-and-socket swivel allows easy positioning for activation by the chin.

Controlflex Ribbon Switch
Press-at-any-point control with nominal finger pressure. Ideal for foot switching.

Controlflex Under-Rug Switching Runner
Requires five pounds of nominal foot pressure. Operates under plywood covered by any sort of tiles.

EMG Switch
This switch makes use of electromyographic (EMG) signals present in a contracting muscle. The EMG switch is a dual-channel device and can use one muscle to replace a single switch or two muscles to replace a dual switch.

Foot Switch
Requires five pounds of nominal foot pressure for activation. User can stand or jump on it! Can be taped or cemented, or can lie loose.

Hand Flexswitch
Switching action occurs when unit is flexed approximately 10 degrees.

Infrared Pickup
Switch is activated by interruption of an infrared beam. Any part of the body is capable of operating the pickup, either by proximity or by interrupting the infrared beam. Particularly useful for persons incapable of precise movements.

Joystick (four micro switches)
Permits directed scanning according to the direction in which it is pushed. Diagonal scanning is also possible. Appropriate for use with communication aids.

Keyboard (expanded)
Keyboard is designed for persons with insufficient coordinated movement to allow efficient use of a normal typewriter. Especially useful for persons with involuntary movements.

LED Sensors
In operation, the optical pointer, when directed at a particular LED within an array, will cause that LED to become bright, thereby showing the user where he or she is pointing. Each LED corresponds to a selection, and when an LED is held on for a short time (acceptance time), the selection is made.

Lever Switch
Light two-way lever action; center off. The lever is pushed or pulled to activate a switch.

Manual Pointer
Permits direct selection activation of communication aids. The photo diode is mounted in a set of plastic, slide-together parts to accommodate various positions of the hand. It can also be mounted to a mouthstick or headstick.

Myoelectric Switch
This switch requires only a slight muscle contraction. An electrode is placed over the muscle site, and a contraction of the muscle produces an electrical signal necessary to activate the switch.

Normally Open Detector Cells
Flat sensing switches in wafer form. Designed to be placed under objects to detect removal.

Optical Headpointer
Permits direct selection activation of communication aids designed with LEDs. This approach permits the individual with good head control to operate the aid. When the optical headpointer is directed at one of the array of lamps, the photo diode in the headpointer senses the LED and activates that location. The headpointer is mounted to a light-weight headband with foam temple pads. Both the headband size and the angle of the optical headpointer are adjustable. It may also be mounted on eyeglass frames.

Pedal Switch
Light pressure on either side of the case. Particularly useful where a part of the body can exert light pressure on two locations reliably.

Pneumatic Pickup
Adjustable pressure on a cushion of plastic material is required for activation. Particularly indicated for persons capable of making relatively precise movements.

Pneumatic Switch
This switch requires sucking or blowing on a tube or pressing an air cushion. Minimal pressure changes are necessary.

Pneumatic Switch
Breath control rather than respiratory control is necessary. Blowing activates one switch, and sucking activates the second switch. An extra 19″ gooseneck is included to extend the mouthpiece if necessary. Extra pneumatic switch tubes (PST-10) are available.

Pneumatic Switch
Light puff or suction on a disposable straw activates the switching mechanism. Particularly useful in situations where breath control is good.

Push Switch
Push switches require a physical movement for activation. The configuration, number of switches, operating movement, and required force need to be consistent with user capabilities.

Radar Pickup
Switch is activated when approached by another object. Since the system detects movement only, it is relatively tolerant of spastic/imprecise movement.

Rocking Lever
Switch is available in both single and dual configurations and with both low and medium forces. It is generally activated with gross hand, arm, or other body part movements, or with a mouthstick or headstick.

Rocking Lever Pneumatic Switch
Light touch of the paddle sends a low-pressure air pulse to a remote pressure switch. It can be used in wet areas since the control portion and tubing are non-electric.

Sound Activated Switch (SAS)
Converts sound level to a switch closure. Sensitivity and acceptance time are adjustable. Can control any device that requires a single control switch.

Spring Wobblestick
These switches can be operated by knocking them in any direction. Ideally suited for gross uncontrolled movement.

Tongue Switch
The control signal is given by the tongue and tongue moisture. The disabled person needs only to touch the contact points of the sensor with the tongue for operation.

Touch Switch
Touch of the skin to the metal rings or disc activates the switch. Very little force or no force is required for activation because it senses a property other than force.

Tongue Switch
Very little force is required for activation. The tongue switch is face-related and may be operated by using the tongue, nose, cheek, or a slight finger movement.

Touch Board
Large touch plates are easily operated by light touch to either pad. Especially useful for persons who can "move" a part of the body over the surface sensor for momentary input.

Wobble Switch
Switch is activated by pushing the ball in any direction. Switch was developed as a convenient means to utilize gross body and head movement for the control of electric devices.

Wobble Switch (single micro switch)
Activated via gross body or head movement from any direction of the switch. It is mounted on a 19″ gooseneck with bracket clamp for easy mounting. Appropriate for row-column and linear scanning of communication aids.

Appendix F
Dedicated Communication Aids

The dedicated communication aids listed in this appendix do not represent an extensive survey of the aids currently available. Rather, they are meant to serve as examples of the categories presented in the text.

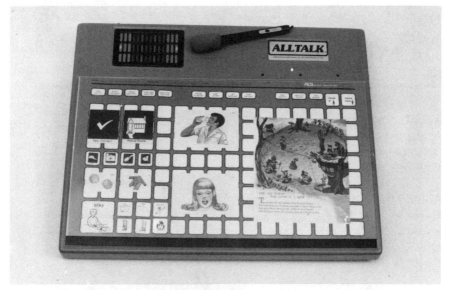

Courtesy of Adaptive Communication Systems.

AllTalk

AllTalk is a human voice output communicator and training aid. AllTalk has 128 programmable locations – anyone's voice may be stored as a message for any given location (AllTalk stores messages on microchips, providing instant retrieval and lasting quality of message reproduction). Environmental noises, music, or any other desired sound may also be stored at any location. AllTalk is completely user programmable. All words, phrases, or sounds may be easily changed at any time by pressing the "program" square and speaking into the microphone. The user may design overlays in any desired manner to correspond to messages programmed. The size of each area of selection is also user-definable. Voice programs may also be stored on any standard cassette player for access at a later time.

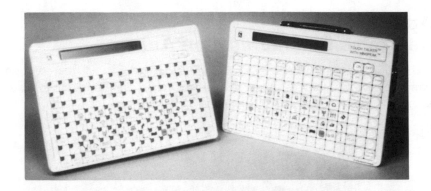

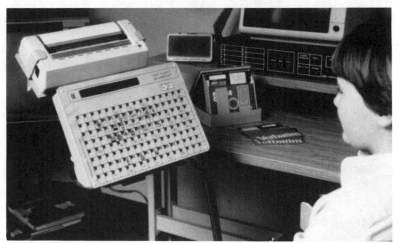

Courtesy of Prentke Romich Co.

Light Talker

The *Light Talker* is a microprocessor-based communication aid with synthesized speech output and a 26,000 character memory. Light Talker operates with either the Express or Minspeak firmware, or both. Minspeak is a concept-based sentence retrieval system; Express is based on levels and locations for storing and retrieving information. Express and Minspeak together provide a fast and effective means of communication. Light Talker has 128 message locations, but the number of locations may be reduced to 32 or to 8 for a smaller number of selections. Light Talker has a built-in correctable display for assembling information to be stored or spoken.

Minspeak I

Minspeak I (or the Express 3 with Minspeak software) is a microprocessor-based communication aid designed around a symbol system unique to the individual user. Minspeak I allows the user to retrieve stored sentences by indicating a small number of symbols. The user may choose from a set of symbols provided with the Minspeak I, or design custom symbols. Symbols may be grouped according to activities of daily living or in any other sequence desired by the user. All words, phrases, and sentences stored in Minspeak I may be entered, changed, or deleted at any time by the user. Synthetic speech output may accompany any sentence constructed. Minspeak I also has a built-in 40-character display and 40-character tape printer.

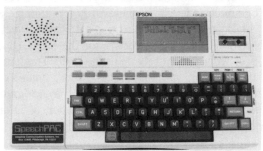

Courtesy of Adaptive Communication Systems.

SpeechPAC/Epson

SpeechPAC/Epson is a portable synthetic voice communicator with a full-sized keyboard, built-in printer, an LCD screen, and a built-in microcassette drive for saving and loading programs. The user types messages on the SpeechPAC keyboard, and messages may then be spoken or directed to the built-in printer. The device can store up to 23,000 characters in memory, giving the user a completely customized voice output. SpeechPAC comes with an abbreviation expansion program called LOLEC, which allows the user to recall messages of up to 250 characters by entering up to four keystrokes. LOLEC and text-to-speech may be mixed at any time and in any combination. A single keystroke instructs the device to print a list of phrase and letter codes in memory. SpeechPAC will operate for up to 20 hours on one battery charge.

VOIS 130

The *VOIS 130* is a portable voice synthesizer for nonvocal individuals. VOIS 130 has a display board with 128 squares. Each square may be represented as a word, a picture, or a symbol. VOIS 130 has four preprogrammed levels — each level may have a separate overlay, or all four levels may be reached from a single master overlay. VOIS 130 has a fifth level which has 118 user programmable locations for selection, and a 4,000 keystroke memory. Words and phrases may be selected, held in memory, and then spoken by VOIS 130, or each word or phrase may be spoken as it is selected.

VOIS 135

VOIS 135 is a voice output communication device with 118 selection locations on each of four programmable levels. The user may program messages or words for each location, or locations may be grouped for larger selection areas. Any symbols or words may be placed on overlays for the VOIS 135, and the organization of symbols or words is entirely up to the user. The four programmable levels may be used to group vocabulary sets (work, home, etc.) or to hold vocabulary sets for a number of users. The user may program spoken messages using phonemes to ensure proper pronunciation of intended words or messages. A keyguard is available for the VOIS 135.

VOIS 140

The *VOIS 140* is a three-digit encoding communication aid with speech output. VOIS 140 contains approximately 986 preprogrammed words, letters, phrases, numbers, and phonemes, and has additional capacity for user-definable words and phrases. The keyboard of the VOIS 140 is a four-by-four matrix that includes numerals 0 through 9 and six operational keys. Messages may be constructed and stored in the VOIS 140's 3,000-keystroke memory and spoken as a group, or each word or phrase may be spoken as it is encoded.

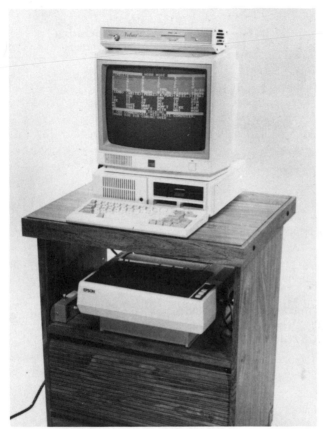

Courtesy of Words+, Inc.

Words+ Living Center III

Words+ Living Center III is a communication system based on the Apple IIe, IIc, or IBM PC microcomputer. *Words+ Living Center III* may be operated by one switch, partial keyboard, or full keyboard. The system provides a means of communication as well as environmental control, drawing, educational, and entertainment functions. The user may produce output at up to 20 words per minute with *Words+ Living Center III.* Output may be displayed on the screen, printed on a printer, or spoken through a speech synthesizer. Use of the *Words+ Living Center III* requires no prior knowledge of computers.

*Source: Bengston, Brandenburg, & Vanderheiden (in press).

Device	USA Manufacturer Distributor	Direct Operating Techniques	Type of Scan
ALLTALK	Adaptive Communication Systems	Direct Selection	
BODAI COMMUNICATOR	Sontek Medical, Inc.	Direct Selection	
CANON COMMUNICATOR MARK 2	Canon USA	Direct Selection	
EXPANDED KEYBOARD MEMOWRITER	Prentke Romich Company	Direct Selection	
EXPRESS 3 standard membrane version	Prentke Romich Company	Direct Selection	
HANDIVOICE 110	Phonic Ear, Inc.	Direct Selection	
PERSONAL COMMUNICATOR	Audiobionics	Direct Selection	
Language Translators	General products	Direct Selection	
Personal Computers (hand-held)	General products (e.g., Sharp, Radio Shack)	Direct Selection	
Personal Computers (portable, lapboard)	General products (e.g., Epson HX-20, Radio Shack Model 100)	Direct Selection	
SAY-IT-ALL	Innocomp	Direct Selection	
SAY-IT-ALL SUPER PLUS	Innocomp	Direct Selection	
SPEAK N' SPELL	Texas Instruments (General product)	Direct Selection	
SPECIAL FRIEND SPEECH PROSTHESIS LCD Model	Shea Products, Inc.	Direct Selection	

Device	USA Manufacturer Distributor	Direct Operating Techniques	Type of Scan
SPEECH AID	Intex Micro Systems Corp.	Direct Selection	
TOUCH TALKER Minspeak Version	Prentke Romich Company	Direct Selection	
TOUCH TALKER EXPRESS 3 Version	Prentke Romich Company	Direct Selection	
TTYs – Portable		Direct Selection	
Typewriters (battery operated)	General products (e.g., Brothers, Canon TypeStar 5)	Direct Selection	
VOCAID	Texas Instruments	Direct Selection	
VOIS 130	Phonic Ear, Inc.	Direct Selection	
VOIS 135	Phonic Ear, Inc.	Direct Selection	
VOIS 140	Phonic Ear, Inc.	Direct Selection	
WORDS+ PORTABLE COMMUNICATOR expanded keyboard version	Words+, Inc.	Direct Selection	
WORDS+ PORTABLE VOICE II expanded keyboard version	Words+, Inc.	Direct Selection	
ACS SPEECH PAC/EPSON – keyboard scan version	Adaptive Communication Systems	Direct Selection & Scan	Row-Group-Item (auditory and visual)
ACS SPEECH PAC/EPSON – scan PAC version	Adaptive Communication Systems	Direct Selection & Scan	Row-Group-Item Directed scan (auditory and visual)
EXPRESS 3 (remote membrane LED version)	Prentke Romich Company	Direct Selection & Scan	Row-Column Directed scan (4–5 switches or joystick)

Device	USA Manufacturer Distributor	Direct Operating Techniques	Type of Scan
FORM-A-PHRASE	Adaptive Communication Systems	Direct Selection & Scan	Linear (of number code)
HANDIVOICE 120	Phonic Ear, Inc.	Direct Selection & Scan	Linear (of number code, auditory and visual)
MINSPEAK 1 (remote membrane LED version)	Prentke Romich Company	Direct Selection & Scan	Row-Column Directed scan (4–5 switches or joystick)
SPECIAL FRIEND SCANNING SPEECH PROSTHESIS	Shea Products, Inc.	Direct Selection & Scan	Row-Column Directed scan (2–5 switches or joystick)
WORDS+ PORTABLE COMMUNICATOR keyboard/external switch version	Words+, Inc.	Direct Selection & Scan	Linear Scan: Morse Code (automatic or manual) Group/Item (alphabet)
WORDS+ PORTABLE VOICE II keyboard/external switch version	Words+, Inc.	Direct Selection & Scan	Linear Scan: Morse Code (automatic or manual) Group/Item (alphabet)
DIAL SCAN	Don Johnson Developmental Equipment	Scan	Linear (automatic)
I COMM	Intex Micro Systems Corp.	Scan	Row-Column
OMNI I	Communications Research Corp.	Scan	Linear (automatic) Row-Column Directed (8-way joystick)
OMNI II	Communications Research Corp.	Scan	Linear (automatic) Row-Column Directed (8-way joystick)

Device	USA Manufacturer Distributor	Direct Operating Techniques	Type of Scan
POSSUM Communicator 16	Possum, Inc.	Scan	Linear (manual & automatic) Directed (2 switches)
POSSUM Communicator 100	Possum, Inc.	Scan	Row Column (manual & automatic) Directed (2–8 switches)
POSSUM LISTEN & LEARN	Possum, Inc.	Scan	Linear (manual & automatic) Directed (2–8 switches)
SCAN WRITER	Zygo Industries, Inc.	Scan	Row-Column Directed scan
TIM	Computers for the Physical Handicapped	Scan	Linear (automatic)
VERSASCAN	Prentke Romich Company	Scan	Linear (manual or automatic)
WORDS+ SCANNING PANEL	Words+, Inc.	Scan	Linear
ZYGO MODEL 16C Communication System	Zygo Industries, Inc.	Scan	Linear (manual or automatic) Directed (2 switches)
ZYGO MODEL 100 Communication System	Zygo Industries, Inc.	Scan	Row-Column Directed (2–5 switches)
Personal Computers (non-portable)	General products (e.g., Apple, IBM)	Direct Selection & Scan (with software and peripherals)	Varies with hardware/software
POSSUM TYPEWRITING SYSTEM	Possum, Inc.	Direct Selection & Scan	Directed (2–8 Switches)
WORDS+ LIVING CENTER (IBM/APPLE)	Words+, Inc.	Direct Selection & Scan	Row-Column with special enhancements

Source: A. Kraat and M. Silver, *Features of Commercially Available Communication Aids*, Prentke Romich Company, 1985.

Appendix G
Selected Dedicated Communication Software

Handicapped Typewriter (Rocky Mountain Software, 214–131 Water Street, Vancouver, B.C., Canada V6B 4M3). Allows the user single-switch interface to achieve letter-by-letter spelling and message retrieval on an enlarged control display. Output options include speech, print, monitor.

Message Maker (Charles Merrill Publishing Co., Columbus, OH 43216). Allows user to type message onto a screen and output it as speech.

Message Maker (Merrill). Allows a user to type a message onto the screen and output it as speech via a scanning technique.

Touch and Speak (Merrill). Allows the user to enter a single keystroke to access a predetermined set of words and phases and generate synthesized speech.

Scan and Speak (Merrill). Allows the user to scan a predetermined set of words, phrases, or pictures and select to generate synthesized speech.

Communication Board Construction Program (Merrill). Allows the clinician to design and print out hardcopy communication board for patients requiring an interim system.

Desk Top (Merrill). Provides the handicapped student the integration of electronic communication, word processing, and a scratch pad for math.

Prometheus Communicator (Prometheus Software, System Support, 5 Devon Street, Lynbrook, NY 11563, 516-599-1416). Allows the user single-switch, letter-by-letter spelling and word retrieval communication through print, speech, and monitor.

Talking Blissapple (Trace Center, University of Wisconsin, S151 Waisman Center, 1500 Highland Avenue, Madison, WI 53705). Allows individuals who use Blissymbolics to use an Apple computer as a talking typewriter with single switch to keyboard interface.

Say It (Schneier Communication Unit, Cerebral Palsy Center, 1603 Court Street, Syracuse, NY 13208). Allows user with single-switch interface to scan (synthesized speech) a series of utterance frames with optional words to complete the utterance.

Words + Living Center III (Words +, Inc, 1125 Steward Court, Suite D., Sunnyvale, CA 94086). Provides user with communication augmentation, some environmental control, and games. Stored words and phrases are used to build messages which can be spoken, printed, or saved to disk. Single-switch or keyboard interface.

Target (Howard Shane, Children's Hospital and Medical Center, Fegan 9, 300 Longwood Ave., Boston, MA 02115). Practice scanning program (visual-stepped, linear, row-column, and directed) with single-switch and joystick interface and variable control display. The program is symbol-empty, and output is displayed on monitor.

Quick Talk (Schneier Communication Unit). Allows spoken output for user with limited ability to use a keyboard. User types number keys to access a personalized dictionary of words and sentences.

Magic Cymbals (Schneier Communication Unit). Allows user with symbol recognition ability (Picsyms and words) and single-switch control to communicate through synthesized speech, print, and monitor.

Talking Word Board (Adaptive Peripherals, 4529 Bagley Avenue North, Seattle, WA 98103). With Unicorn Board, Echo Speech Synthesizer, and Adaptive Firmware Card, allows the user to speak messages that are prepared letter-by-letter or retrieved. The system operates with a symbol-free format.

Talking Unicorn Board (Adaptive Peripherals). Requires the same equipment as Talking Word Board. Allows user to control Apple computer via the expanded Unicorn Board. The TUB program provides spoken output of expanded keyboard commands.

Talking Unicorn Board (Adaptive Peripherals). Requires the same equipment as the Talking Word Board. Allows the user to control the Apple computer through scanning modes with the commands spoken by the synthesizer.

Predictive Linguistics Program (Adaptive Peripherals). Requires Apple IIe with 128K and Adaptive Firmware Card. Allows the user to enhance communication and writing speed by a system of word retrieval based on "guessing." As the user begins to spell a word, the computer "guesses" the word intended. Up to nine words are offered as guesses.

Source: Beukelmen, 1986.

References

Alpert, C. (1980). Procedures for determining the optimal nonspeech mode with the autistic child. In R. L. Schiefelbusch (Ed.), *Nonspeech language and communication: Analysis and intervention* (pp. 389–421). Austin, TX: PRO-ED.

ASHA (1980). Non-speech communication: A position paper. *ASHA, 22,* 267–272.

Balick, S., Spiegel, D., & Greene, G. (1976). Mime in language therapy and clinician training. *Archives of Physical Medical Rehabilitation, 57,* 35–38.

Bengston, D., Brandenburg, S., & Vanderheiden, G. (in press). *Non-vocal communication resource book* (rev. ed.). San Diego, CA: College Hill Press.

Beukelman, D. (1986). *Dedicated communication software listing.* Presentation at the American-Speech-Language Hearing Computer Conference, Orlando, Florida.

Beukelman, D., & Yorkston, K. (1977). A communication system for the severely dysarthric speaker with an intact language system. *Journal of Speech and Hearing Disorders, 42,* 265–270.

Beukelman, D. R., & Yorkston, K. M. (1982). Communication interaction of adult communication augmentation system use. *Topics in Language Disorders, 2,* 39–54.

Beukelman, D., Yorkston, K., & Dowden, P. (1985). *Communication augmentation: A casebook of clinical management.* San Diego, CA: College Hill Press.

Blissymbolics. Blissymbolics Communication Institute, 350 Rumsey Road, Toronto, Ontario M4G 1R8, Canada.

Buzolich, M. J. (1981, April). *Assessment and training methodology for the adult user of a vocal output communication device.* Paper presented at the California Speech-Language-Hearing Association, San Francisco, CA.

Carrier, J. K. (1976). Application of a nonspeech language system with the severely handicapped. In R. L. Schiefelbusch (Ed.), *Communication assessment and intervention strategies* (pp. 523–547). Austin, TX: PRO-ED.

Chapman, R. S., & Miller, J. F. (1980). Analyzing language and communication in the child. In R. L. Schiefelbusch (Ed.), *Nonspeech language and communication: Analysis and intervention* (pp. 159–196). Austin, TX: PRO-ED.

Chen, L. Y. (1971). Manual communication by combined alphabet and gestures. *Archives of Physical Medical Rehabilitation, 52,* 381–384.

Chial, M. R. (1984). Glossary of microcomputer terms. In A. Schwartz (Ed.), *Handbook of microcomputer applications in communication disorders* (pp. 275–309). San Diego, CA: College Hill Press.

Cohen, C., & Shane, H. (1982). An overview of augmentative communication. In N. H. Lass, L. M. McReynolds, J. L. Northern, & D. E. Yoder (Eds.), *Speech, Language, and Hearing: Vol. II* (pp. 875–889). Philadelphia: W. B. Saunders.

Creak, M. (1961). Schizophrenic syndrome in childhood: Progress report of a working party. *Cerebral Palsy Bulletin, 3,* 501–504.

Darley, F. L., Aronson, A. E., & Brown, J. R. (1975). *Motor speech disorders.* Philadelphia: W. B. Saunders.

Dartnall, N. A. (1980). Manual sign training as an aid to language learning by autistic children. *Journal of Childhood Communication Disorders, 4,* 56–57.

DeRuyter, F., & David, D. S. (1982, November). *Transitional and permanent usage of augmentative communication with the head-injured.* Paper presented at the American-Speech-Language-Hearing Association, Toronto, Canada.

Estabrooks, N., & Walsh, M. (1985). Unpublished paper on head injury and augmentative communication.

Fenn, G., & Rowe, J. A. (1975). An experiment in manual communication. *British Journal of Disorders of Communication, 10,* 3–16.

Ferrier, L. J., & Shane, H. C. (1983). A description of non-speaking population under consideration for augmentative communication systems. In *Advances in Mental Handicap Research* (vol. 2, pp. 95–137). New York: John Wiley & Sons.

Fulwiller, R. L., & Fouts, R. S. (1976). Acquisition of American sign language by a noncommunicating autistic child. *Journal of Autism and Childhood Schizophrenia, 6,* 43–51.

Grove, N. M. (1976). Conditions resulting in physical disabilities. In *Teaching individuals with physical and multiple disabilities.* Columbus: Merrill Publishing.

Guess, D., Sailor, W., & Baer, D. (1978). Children with limited language. In R. L. Schiefelbusch (Ed.), *Language intervention strategies.* Austin, TX: PRO-ED.

Guess, D., Sailor, W., & Baer, D. (1976). *Functional speech and language training for the retarded.* Lawrence, KS: H & H Enterprises.

Harris, D., & Vanderheiden, G. (1980a). Enhancing the development of communicative interaction. In R. L. Schiefelbusch (Ed.), *Nonspeech language and communication: Analysis and intervention* (pp. 227–258). Austin, TX: PRO-ED.

Harris, D., & Vanderheiden, G. C. (1980b). Augmentative communication techniques. In R. L. Schiefelbusch (Ed.), *Nonspeech language and communication: Analysis and intervention* (pp. 259–302). Austin, TX: PRO-ED.

Harris-Vanderheiden, D., & Vanderheiden, G. C. (1977). Basic considerations in the development of communicative and interactive skills for non-vocal severely handicapped children. In E. Sontag, J. Smith, & N. Certo (Eds.), *Education programming for the severely and profoundly handicapped* (pp. 323–334). Reston, VA: Council for Exceptional Children.

Kahn, J. (1977). A comparison of manual and oral language training with mute retarded children. *Mental Retardation, 16,* 21–23.

Kanner, L. (1943). Autistic disturbances of affective contact. *Nervous Child, 2,* 217–250.

Kent, L. R. (1974). *Language acquisition program for the retarded or multiply impaired.* Champaign, IL: Research Press.

Kiernan, C. (1983). The use of nonvocal communication techniques with autistic individuals. *Journal of Child Psychology and Psychiatry, 24,* 339–375.

Levett, L. M. (1969). A method of communication for non-speaking, severely subnormal children. *British Journal of Disorders of Communication, 4,* 64–66.

Light, P. H., & Remington, R. E. (1978). *Approaches to language intervention: Symbol utilization by non-verbal autistic children.* Paper presented to the Conference of the Development Section of the British Psychological Society, Nottingham.

McDonald, E. T. (1980). Early identification and treatment of children at risk for speech development. In R. L. Schiefelbusch (Ed.), *Nonspeech language and communication: Analysis and intervention* (pp. 27–80). Austin, TX: PRO-ED.

McDonald, E. T. (1976). Language foundations. In G. C. Vanderheiden & K. Grilley (Eds.), *Non-vocal communication techniques and aids for the severely physically handicapped.* Austin, TX: PRO-ED.

McDonald, E. T., & Schultz, A. R. (1973). Communication boards for cerebral-palsied children. *Journal of Speech and Hearing Disorders, 38,* 73–78.

Miller, A., & Miller, E. E. (1973). Cognitive developmental training with elevated boards and sign language. *Journal of Autism and Childhood Schizophrenia, 3,* 65–85.

Moore, B., Haynes, J., & Laing, C. (1978). *Introduction to symptoms and terminology.* Springfield, IL: Charles C. Thomas.

Murphy, J. W., & Cook, A. M. (1975). Limitations of augmentative communication systems in progressive neurological diseases. In C. Brubaker (Ed.), *Proceedings of the Eighth Annual Conference on Rehabilitation Technology.* Washington, DC: RESNA.

Musselwhite, C. R., & St. Louis, K. W. (1982). *Communication programming for the severely handicapped.* San Diego, CA: College Hill Press.

Mysak, E. E. (1963). Dysarthria and oropharyngeal reflexology: A review. *Journal of Speech and Hearing Disorders, 28,* 252–260.

National Institute of Handicapped Research (1984). *Digest of data on persons with disabilities.* Mathematica Policy Research, Inc., 600 Maryland Avenue, S.W., Washington, DC 20024.

National Institute of Neurological and Communicative Disorders and Stroke (1976). *Neurological and communicative disorders—estimated numbers and cost.* DHEW Publication No. (NIH) 77-152 (rev.). Washington, DC: Author.

Offir, C. W. (1976). Visual speech: Their fingers do the talking. *Psychology Today, 10*(1), 72–78.

Proceedings, BEH Conference on Communication Aids for the Non-Vocal Severely Physically Handicapped Persons (1976, December). Alexandria, Virginia.

Reichle, J., & Yoder, D. E. (1985). Communication board use in severely handicapped learners. *Language, Speech, and Hearing Services in Schools, 16,* 1–11.

Rimland, B. (1964). *Infantile autism.* New York: Appleton, Century.

Ritvo, E. R., & Freeman, B. J. (1978). National Society for Autistic Children definition of the syndrome of autism. *Journal of Autism and Childhood Schizophrenia, 8,* 162–167.

Rutter, M. (1966). Prognosis: Psychotic children in adolescent and early adult life. In J. K. Wing (Ed.), *Early childhood autism: Clinical, educational, and social aspects* (pp. 83–100). London: Pergamon Press.

Shane, H. C. (1980). Approaches to assessing the communication of people who are nonoral. In R. L. Schiefelbusch (Ed.), *Nonspeech language and communication.* Austin, TX: PRO-ED.

Shane, H. C. (1979). Approaches to communication training with the severely handicapped. In R. L. York & E. Edgar (Eds.), *Teaching the severely handicapped, Vol. IV* (pp. 155–179). Columbus, OH: Special Press.

Shane, H. C., & Bashir, A. S. (1980). Election criteria for the adoption of an augmentative communication system: Preliminary considerations. *Journal of Speech and Hearing Disorders, 45,* 408–415.

Shane, H. C., & Yoder, D. E. (1981). Delivery of augmentative communication services: The role of the speech-language pathologist. *Language, Speech, and Hearing in the Schools, 12,* 211–215.

Silverman, F. L. (1980). *Communication for the speechless.* Englewood Cliffs, NJ: Prentice-Hall.

Silverman, F. H. (1977). Criteria for assessing therapy outcome in speech pathology and audiology. *Journal of Speech and Hearing Research, 20,* 5–20.

Sitver, M., & Kraat, A. (1982, November). *Amyotrophic lateral sclerosis (ALS) and augmentative communication.* Paper presented at the American Speech-Language-Hearing Association, Toronto.

Skelly, M., Donaldson, R. C., & Fust, R. S. (1973). *Glossectomee speech rehabilitation.* Springfield, IL: Charles C. Thomas.

Song, A. (1979). Acquisition and use of Blissymbols by severely mentally retarded adolescents. *Mental Retardation, 17,* 253–255.

Topper, S. T. (1975). Gesture language for a non-verbal severely retarded male. *Mental Retardation, 13*(1), 30–31.

Vanderheiden, G. C., & Grilley, K. (Eds.). (1976). *Non-vocal communication techniques and aids for the severely physically handicapped.* Austin, TX: PRO-ED.

Vanderheiden, G. C., & Harris-Vanderheiden, D. H. (1976). Communication techniques and aids for the nonvocal severely handicapped. In L. Lloyd (Ed.), *Communication assessment and intervention strategies.* Austin, TX: PRO-ED.

Vanderheiden, G. C., & Lloyd, L. L. (in press). Communication systems and their components. In S. Blackstone (Ed.), *Augmentative communication: An introduction.* Washington, DC: American Speech-Language-Hearing Association.

Vicker, B. (Ed.). (1974). *Nonoral communication project 1964/1973.* Iowa City, IA: Campus Stores.

Yorkston, K., & Karlan, G. (1986). *Evaluation assessment procedures in augmentative communication: An introduction.* Orlando, FL: American Speech-Language-Hearing Association.

Wilson, P. S., Goodman, L., & Wood, R. K. (1975). *Manual language for the child without language: A behavioral approach for teaching the exceptional child.* Hartford, CT: Department of Mental Retardation Developmental Team.

Yarrow, L., Klein, R., Lomonaco, S., & Morgan, G. (1975). Cognitive and motivational development in early childhool. In B. Friedlander, G. Sterritt, & G. Kirk (Eds.), *Exceptional infant, Vol. 3.* New York: Brunner-Mazel.

Maggie Sauer is a speech-language pathologist at the Trace Center at the University of Wisconsin—Madison, Waisman Center. She is presently the clinician for the Communication Development Program, a community-based program that provides training for and evaluation of nonspeaking children and adults. She is also involved in information services at the Trace Center, educating professionals and individuals about augmentative communication and training techniques.

Howard Shane is Director of the Communication Enhancement Clinic at The Children's Hospital, Boston. He is a widely published author of numerous books, chapters, and articles dealing with augmentative and alternative communication. In addition, he has served on a number of professional committees directly related to this topic.